BIOETHICS AT THE CROSSROAD OF RELIGIONS:
Thoughts on the Foundations of Bioethics in Christianity and Islam

BIOETHICS AT THE CROSSROAD OF RELIGIONS:

Thoughts on the Foundations of Bioethics in Christianity and Islam

Antoine Tarabay

Foreword by Cardinal George Pell

Connor Court Publishing

Connor Court Publishing Pty Ltd

Copyright © Antoine Tarabay 2015

ALL RIGHTS RESERVED. This book contains material protected under International and Federal Copyright Laws and Treaties. Any unauthorised reprint or use of this material is prohibited. No part of this book may be reproduced or transmitted in any form or by any means, electronic or mechanical, including photocopying, recording, or by any information storage and retrieval system without express written permission from the publisher.

PO Box 224W
Ballarat VIC 3350
sales@connorcourt.com
www.connorcourt.com

ISBN: 9781925138672 (pbk.)

Cover design by Ian James

Printed in Australia

Dedication

*Ave Maria, my Holy Mother in this earthly life,
you inspired me with your love, and
through your intercessions, I am blessed.*

*To the Church my mater et maestra,
to my family the Lebanese Maronite Order,
and to my beloved parents and siblings.
Without you, I would not be here today
living my deep faith,*

*and be
bestowed with the grace of being a member in
the mystic body of our Lord, Jesus Christ,
and now, chosen to be a shepherd
tending to the Lord's flock here in this land of the Southern Cross.*

CONTENTS

Foreword by Cardinal George Pell ix

Acknowledgements xi

Introduction xii

Part One: 'Man' Creature of God

1. Bioethics and the concept of Man in Catholicism 3

2. Bioethics and the concept of Man in Islam 23

   Postscript: Convergences and Divergences 44

Part Two: The Significance of Human Sexuality

3. Bioethics and Sexuality: The Catholic Perspective 51

4. Bioethics and Sexuality: The Islamic Perspective 68

   Postscript: Convergences and Divergences 81

Part Three: The Significance of Human Corporeality

5. Bioethics and Corporeality in Catholicism 91

6. Bioethics and Corporeality in Islam 109

   Postscript: Convergences and Divergences 125

Part Four: Health and Sickness: Ethical Principles

7. Bioethics, Health and Sickness in Catholicism 133

8. Bioethics, Health and Sickness in Islam 145

    Postscript: Convergences and Divergences 158

    Conclusion 161

    Bibliography 163

    About the author 173

    Glossary...175

Foreword

by Cardinal George Pell

quondam Archbishop of Sydney

Prefect of the Secretariat for the Economy

It has been said that one's image of God determines how one treats other people.

In the Catholic Christian tradition, there are some key foundations which determine our entire approach to God and man.

First, as we learn in *Genesis*, all humans are made "in the image of God." This means that we can learn something about God by studying His creatures, man and woman, who have a heart for tender loving, a will for freely choosing, and a mind for rational understanding.

Then, as to God Himself, we believe in His Fatherhood. "I believe in God the Father almighty, Creator of heaven and earth." God is not some remote Supreme Being, alien to us and the world. Rather, He is our loving Father; and through human relations, we can come closer to God and deepen in our understanding of Him.

Thirdly, God is *Logos* – Reason – and the source of reason. The Divine Wisdom cannot do or command anything contrary to reason. He may do or mandate things above the limits of human wisdom, but He can never command what is inherently absurd or unreasonable. This has major implications for morality.

Finally, we have the great declaration of St John, the Beloved Disciple: "God is love." It is His very nature to love. He cannot hate what He has made. All that He made is good, very good indeed, as *Genesis* tells us.

It is sin – violation of God's commands – that disfigures human beings. But if we respect our bodies and souls as they have been made, to make us images of God our loving Father, then indeed we will be both good and blessed, as we fulfil God's plan for human life here below, in preparation for the eternal life.

I think that many Christians take these foundations for granted, and presume that Moslems equally accept them. Do they know that while all four foundations are in the Christian Bible, not only are they absent from the *Koran* but they are *denied* by Islam?

I realise, of course, that such ancient foundations, however necessary, do not answer all the complicated and delicate ethical questions that confront us in the face of modern bio-technology. However, unless we are clear about our foundations, we will be off track even before we begin to search for where the answers lie.

I commend this study of Maronite Bishop, Antoine-Charbel Tarabay, comparing and contrasting Catholic and Islamic approaches to the foundations of bioethics. Bishop Tarabay's background in the Middle East, his education in Western Europe, and his career as parish priest and educator in Australia, have furnished him with a rare intellectual, linguistic and religious culture and experience to tackle this pressing subject of inter-religious bioethics in the modern world.

Acknowledgements

I am heartily thankful to my supervisor, Rev. Fr. Maurizio Faggioni EFO, who directed my research and carried it to its conclusion, and for his meticulous assistance and his precious observations.

I would like to show my gratitude to Rev. Fr. Maurice Borrmans who agreed to accompany and guide me from the outset of my research journey.

It is an honour for me to thank Cardinal George Pell, former Archbishop of Sydney, for his contribution to the Australian publication. He is a role model, and a source of inspiration for the Catholic Church in Australia.

Lastly, I offer my regards and blessings to all of those who supported me in any respect during the completion of this project. You have helped me to realise my aspiration of seeing the publication of this book.

Introduction

The advancements achieved in medical research over the last 50 years, and the increasingly important place it plays in social and individual life, has had numerous repercussions across many domains. The positive results of these advances are evident, and justify continuing this research to safeguard human life. However, the risks are also undeniable when measured against the prodigal conquests of science, and the immense power that individuals wield with respect to their own lives.

Every living being, possessing as it does, the instinct to preservation and conservation of life, should be inspired with respect for human life. Life is of great value to the human person, yet, good as it is, earthly life is not an absolute value. However, the existence of ideal tendencies in human nature towards *good, beauty and truth,* calls for the founding of norms that regulate human behaviour. The diverse religious beliefs which provide an answer, each in its own manner to these distinct needs of 'man,' seem to be in accordance when professing a respect for life, more or less generalised.

With the above in mind, a comparative bioethical study of the Catholic and Islamic faiths is presented here, with a particular focus on interreligious bioethics. The inviolability of the right to life for an innocent human being is a sign and a requirement of the inviolability of human life itself. The Catholic and Islam faiths clearly call for respect for human life, yet each religion does so according to its own doctrinal, theological and anthropological concepts.

Modern progress in research in the biological and medical sciences, and their application to human beings, has become the subject of numerous studies, and even genuine concern. Violations against basic human rights, with a particular emphasis on biomedical experimentation, have led to the awakening of an international conscience, and have been behind the development of the ethical thought known as *bioethics*. Several definitions have been presented for this relatively new discipline; some are speculative, while others attempt to give a practical dimension to theoretical concepts.

In the infancy of the discipline, the *Encyclopaedia of Bioethics* (Reich, 1978) defined bioethics as,

> The systematic study of human behaviour in the context of the life sciences and health care, whereby such behaviour comes to be examined in light of values and moral principles. (p. xix)

This definition became more explicit when pertaining to ethical differentiation in the 1995 edition:

> Bioethics is the methodical study of the moral dimensions – including moral vision, decisions, behaviour and politics – of life sciences and healthcare, utilising a variety of ethical methodologies in an inter-disciplinary setting.

The above definition views bioethics as a form of practical knowledge. It studies human biomedicine, and determines the ethical criteria capable of orienting and guiding it. With this perspective, bioethics does not manifest itself as a new form of ethics, but rather as a dimension of it.

In this light, Sgreccia (1994) states that:

> Bioethics is a part of moral philosophy that determines whether it is licit or not to intervene in the life of man, particularly when related to the practice and development of medical and biological sciences. (p. 51)

Lega (1991) concurs with Scarpelli, and views bioethics as a component of that larger ethical school of thought that examines the way in which humankind is to regard life.

The aim of bioethics then, is to confront the new challenges faced by society in a manner that respects the value and dignity of life of every human being in their totality. These challenges are in fact the result of medical and research practices that aim to remedy the suffering and distress of those who have been struck by disease or handicap, but which also expose human life to abuse and danger. Medical researchers must question their technological progress and research advances that in turn threaten the fundamental value and dignity of every human being. Contemporary medical practices must refer to medical ethics with respect to those practices that surpass its deontological code. The ethics of the medical and health care professions are, generally speaking, a reflection of the issues raised by medical science and healthcare practices, starting with general principles and the values that ought to be a guide to every act affecting human life.

If the study of bioethics consists of constructing a bridge between the science of life and moral values, then bioethics is a discipline that comprises ethics and medical deontology. When taking the epistemological viewpoint, bioethics comprises three categories of thought. *General bioethics* deals with fundamental ethics and discourse relating to the values and the original principles of medical ethics. *Specialist bioethics* examines specific medical practices that are included within the overall area of general bioethics. *Clinical bioethics* focuses on the discussion and examination of particular cases of medical practice (Sgreccia, 1994).

This comparative study is undertaken in the context of *general bioethics*. Questions of *specialist bioethics* will be addressed in future publications.

When approaching this comparative study of Catholicism and Islam, one must put aside any political and religious prejudices, and consider only the theological facts of each faith and their application to bioethics. As such, this comparative study aims to highlight the ethical values common to the two faiths, their stance on those practices that present a bioethical dilemma, and clarify the differences in thought between Catholicism and Islam.

In brief, this study will tentatively consider how the Catholic and Islamic faiths respond to the wider options in healthcare which exist today due to continual innovation in medical research, and subsequent changes in medical practices.

At the core of this bioethical discussion, is the individual experience in Catholicism or Islam that a person undertakes when faced with a bioethical dilemma. As such, this study will explore the anthropological foundations of bioethics. The concept of human life being the creation of God will be introduced, and then we will discuss the essential dignities and non-alienable rights possessed by a human being. The concept of humans as sexual beings will also be explored, as will the manner in which sexuality, as a part of human nature, is manifested through the human body, and the importance of this act in shaping each person's values with respect to physical life. The discussion in this first book is intended to bring a deeper *sense of human values* to the scientific fields of medicine and biomedicine, highlighting the understanding of 'man,' sexuality, corporeality and healthcare in an interreligious ethical context.

With the advances in and progression of biological and medical sciences, a renewed awareness of ethical values seems necessary. Nevertheless, the concerns that are associated with bioethics relate to the most fundamental human rights, and respect for each individual being and their dignity throughout each stage of the life cycle – from conception, to old age and to natural death. Hence the question is posed: Is it now a necessity that Catholicism and Islam collaborate on bioethical matters, for the benefit and respect of humanity?

This study was written between 1996 and 1999, as part of a larger doctorate thesis titled *Bioéthique Catholique et Bioéthique Musulmane: étude d'éthique comparée en vue d'une bioéthique interreligieuse*. Although encouraged by thesis supervisors and the author's own students at the Holy Spirit University Kaslik, the earlier publication of this work was not possible due to the author's vocational commitment and service to the Maronite Catholic Church in both Lebanon and Australia. This aside, the publication still remains of benefit for a niche audience interested in bioethics within an interreligious context. The original thesis was completed in French, and it is important to note that some of the quoted references have been translated by the author from Italian, French or Arabic, if no English translation was available.

Within the available resources, this study will explore the anthropological foundations and particular questions of bioethics in the Catholic Church and Islamic faith. Furthermore, it is anticipated that this study will lead to further comprehensive research into bioethics. This discussion is not in the least an attempt to resolve the complexity of the issues that surround bioethics in an interreligious context. This is, rather, a discussion which aims to provide clarity to questions of bioethical concern, and widen the possibility of dialogue between the Catholic Church and Islam.

The main question of the anthropological foundations of bioethics is answered in terms of the human being as a creature who exists in this world. Both the Catholic Church and Islam have distinct frames of reference. These explicitly and implicitly define the scope within which bioethical reason operates to shape a normative content. As such:

> A bioethical reflection that aims to remain human and humanizing, in the elaboration of its moral criteria, must originate from man as a person: in fact, the human person is a value that is fundamental and transcendent, intangible and normative, whether in the ethical reflection or in its practice that aims at remaining completely human and moral. (Frattallone 1994, p.714)

The above notion of the human being as an "inviolable subject", establishes the significance and value of human life, and the ability to identify "ethical subjects."

If bioethics leads to an ethics of life which can only be authentic with an adequate vision of the human being, then morality must presuppose anthropology, and not vice versa. Morality is then to be regarded as the practical aspect of anthropology, and the same can be said for bioethics (Bellino, 1997). The first examination does not concern medical interventions, but, rather, the value of the human person. Consequently, human reality cannot be treated as a means, but rather as an end and an absolute value. Therefore, it is necessary to first explore the relationship between anthropology and bioethics. The question then is how the Catholic and Islamic faiths understand the anthropological foundations of bioethics.

This book will present a comparison of the two anthropological models found in Catholicism and Islam. The anthropological aspects of human creation, sexuality, the human body and health will be explored as presented in the Bible, in conjunction with the *Magisterium*, to highlight the position of Catholicism. The Islamic viewpoint of the same anthropological concepts will then be presented according to the Koran, and other teachings in the *Shari'a*. To ensure an objective comparison, each religious perspective will be presented according to their own religious authorities and scholars.

The core question of whether or not an interreligious anthropology is necessary for the elaboration of interreligious bioethics will be explored in this book. However, the anthropological foundations of interreligious bioethics are strictly related to the core subject that shapes the way of thinking and acting in bioethics.

Part One

'Man': Creature of God

Introduction

As creatures brought into existence by the voluntary act of God, 'man' is a divine creation in Catholicism and Islam. 'Man' in the theological tradition of the monotheistic religions, is "the king and the masterpiece of creation" (Masson 1976, p. 199). Part One aims to establish the anthropological concept of 'man' in Catholicism and Islam, thus enabling a comparative interreligious bioethics.

In addition to the Bible, as the primary reference source of Catholicism, reference will be made to the official magisterial documents of the Catholic Church. They include the Church's contemporary Pastoral Constitution, *Gaudium et Spes* (*Vatican II*), the *Catechism of the Catholic Church*, and the Magisterium of Pope John Paul II.

For Islam, the *Shari'a*, in particular the Koran, and other additional sources will be referenced. They include *Reflexions sur le Coran (Reflections upon the Koran)* (Talbi and Bucaille, 1989), which examines Koranic anthropology whilst asserting the privileged and unique vocation of 'man' in Islam. Al-Naggar (1996), discusses the Islamic concept of 'man' in *Mabda' al-insan (The Principles of Man)* and *Qimat al-insan (The Value of Man)*. Al-Buti (1992) in *Manhag al-hadara al-insaniya (Method of the Human Civilisation in the Koran)*, looks at the roles and responsibilities of the Koranic 'man.'

The anthropological comparison between Catholicism and Islam, will however, be confined to Biblical and Koranic references to 'man'.

1

Bioethics and the Concept of 'Man' in Catholicism

In the Catholic theological tradition, creation is based on a principal belief: the human person, like any other creature or reality in this world, was created by God. Human beings then, do not come into existence simply because of natural evolution, but are in fact God's "favourite creature" entrusted with a spiritual vocation that is beyond the physical world. God created 'man' and brought him into His intimate domain, calling him to become His interlocutor. Nevertheless, *personalist bioethics* in Catholicism is based on the premise that the human being is perceived as an end, not a means. This reality is reflected in the Bible, in particular the Book of Genesis, and is developed in the contemporary teaching of the Magisterium.

'Man' in the Catholic theological tradition

Biblical theology regards 'man' as being exclusively created in the image of God. Instead of confining itself within a natural and enclosed world, Biblical theology opens the scene to the divine dimensions of history, a history which has God as its principal actor: God who has created 'man' and to save him has become 'man' Himself. In this sense, once anthropology is connected to Catholic theology it becomes inseparable from Christology. Accordingly, the historical context of 'man' in the Bible presents two facets – the 'old man', who has sinned in Adam, and then the 'new man' redeemed in Jesus Christ (Koch, 1967).

The creation of man and woman according to the Bible

The creation of man and woman has an important position, if not the central one, within the creative act of God (Colzani, 1988). God the Creator, on whom 'man' and the universe depends, manifests Himself as a living and personal God. Before God, 'man' in his being is fashioned from the dust of the earth. What is remarkable in the creation story is that God *"has created everything for man,"* (*Vatican II Council* 1966, pp. 1034, 1046 and 1070). While creating the universe, God had the creation of 'man' in mind.

In the Book of Genesis, the story of 'man's' creation is presented in two different ways. The first, being an objective perspective, in which:

> God said, 'Let us make man in our own image, in the likeness of ourselves...' God created man in the image of himself, in the image of God he created him, male and female he created them. (Gen 1:26-27)

An alternative concept provides a subjective point of view, where:

> Yahweh God shaped man from the soil of the ground and blew the breath of life into his nostrils, and man became a living being. (Gen 2:7)

The reference to *living being* implies a living person, capable of entering into a relationship with God, and thus defines the true purpose of 'man' (Grelot, 1973). Furthermore:

> Yahweh God said, 'It is not right that the man should be alone. I shall make him a helper.'...Then, Yahweh God made the man fall into a deep sleep. And, while he was asleep, he took one of his ribs and closed the flesh up again forthwith. Yahweh God fashioned the rib he had taken from the man into a woman, and brought her to the man. And the man said: This one at last is bone of my bones and flesh of my

flesh! She is to be called Woman because she was taken from Man. (Gen 2:18-23)

The first text is admittedly concise and lacking all traces of subjectivity. It presents the objective facts and reality when it conveys the creation of 'man' followed with the first benediction (Gen 1:28). The second account of creation however, is presented subjectively, where man was created separately. From the moment God created woman, God referred to man as *ish*, and woman as *ishsha* (Pope John Paul II, 1985).

The first text (Gen 1:26-27), came chronologically after the second text (Gen 2:7; Gen 2:18-23) . The origin of the second text is thought to be much more ancient, and is called "Yahwist", so named chiefly because it often refers to God as *Yahweh*. When comparing the two texts, it appears that the later, originating in the Priestly tradition, provides a more mature image of God and 'man' (Pope John Paul II, 1985).

God the Creator manifested His love for the first time through the act of creation. Created from nothing, 'man' as creature is entirely indebted to God for his existence (Durable, 1960). Furthermore, the following characteristics of 'man's' creation can be ascertained. They are:

1. 'Man' is above all the image of God, whether male or female, and created after the visible world. "Even though he has a direct connection to this world, the Biblical story has no mention of his resemblance to the rest of the creatures, but only to God" (Pope John Paul II 1985, p. 34).

2. God acts through special intervention to form the bodies of the first man and woman. Pope John Paul II (1985, p. 34) adds that "they are not created through natural succession, but the Creator seems to mark

a pause before calling them to existence, as if He is internally deliberating to make a decision: Let us make man in our own image, in the likeness of ourselves ... (Gen 1:26)."

3. The story of God's creation and intervention on earth asserts that God did not create the body of 'man' ex nihilo, that is, from nothing. The second text of creation states that God used existing material, "the dust of the earth," to form man, and "the man's rib" to create woman (Koch 1967, pp. 65-66). This account of the creation of woman is not an attempt to specify where she came from but rather who she is, that is, a being equal to man in nature and dignity. God demonstrates why woman is, amongst all other creatures, the sole match that completes man in the most appropriate way.

4. The personification of 'man' in Adam, happened when he received the spirit of life directly from God. This is what differentiates human beings from all other living creatures. 'Man's existence is due to the spirit of life from the breath by God, enabling 'man' to become a living soul that is an independent being and at the same time a dependant being on God (Leon-Dufour, 1981).

The Biblical view of 'man's' creation can be considered as the foundation for the concept of *mediate animation*, which is one school of thought within Catholicism regarding the moment the rational soul is present in a human being. This concept will be elaborated at a later stage. The historical perspective of human creation emphasises a further two components which we meet in Biblical anthropology: fertility and the relationship of 'man' with the world.

Fertility

According to the Book of Genesis, the biological difference between man and woman is linked to fertility, and thus justifies human existence in society. To the statement, "Yahweh God said, 'It is not right that the man should be alone...' " (Gen 2:18), one must add the notion of one sex complementing the other in a reciprocating relationship to enable fertility, and thus "God blessed them, saying to them, 'Be fruitful, multiply, fill the earth and subdue it.' " (Gen 1:28)

This commandment does not render sexual activity a 'sacred' act, but makes it a necessary component of the human condition. By saying "be fruitful," God blesses sexual activity as an attribute of 'man,' who has been made in His image and thus makes 'man' a sacred being. In this way, the Book of Genesis marks the will of God who wishes that man and woman live out their love within a communion of life and sanctity (Colzani, 1988; Brugues, 1991).

Relation of 'man' with the world

It is evident from Genesis (2:15), that God has placed 'man' in this world to undertake a role in His creation, which is to "cultivate and take care of it" as his custodian. God in fact wanted Adam to assert his sovereignty over the animals by giving him authority to name them, and

> So from the soil Yahweh God fashioned all the wild animals and all the birds of heaven. These he brought to the man to see what he would call them; each one was to bear the name the man would give it. (Gen 2:19)

It can then be ascertained that the earth is not to be divinised, but rather to be dominated. Furthermore, there is a duty to work and to obey God, and carry out God's plans for the world. God's plan includes 'man' observing the seventh day as a day of rest. Thus, man has a duty to work and to rest.

The Biblical text highlights the extent and depth of superiority God has bestowed to 'man', and is seen through the authority 'man' has over the earth and its creatures. It is about 'the domination over earth and every living being," as referenced in the Book of Wisdom below:

> God of our ancestors, Lord of mercy,
> who by your word have made the universe,
> and in your wisdom have fitted human beings
> to rule the creatures that you have made,
> to govern the world in holiness and saving justice
> and in honesty of soul to dispense fair judgement. (Wis 9: 1-3)

In the Book of Psalms, the authority and dominant role given to 'man' is seen to be a reflection of the glory and honour received from the Creator. The psalmist said:

> You [God] made him lord of the works of your hands,
> put all things under his feet,
> sheep and cattle, all of them,
> and even the wild beasts,
> birds in the sky, fish in the sea,
> when he makes his way across the ocean.
> Yahweh our Lord,
> how majestic your name throughout the world! (Ps 8:6-9)

In sum, the Biblical revelation presents the human person as being created in the image of God. The *Catechism of the Catholic Church* (1995) states that man and woman were "created to serve and to love God and to offer Him the whole creation" (358). This revelation is later actualised through Christ, as the Word of God becomes flesh, making every believer a living part of His mystical body, and:

> So for anyone who is in Christ, there is a new creation: the
> old order is gone and a new being is there to see. (2 Cor 5:17)

'Man' in the contemporary Magisterium

The Biblical account of the creation and role of 'man' establishes the foundation of Catholic anthropology, and is thus expanded in the Magisterium. This anthropology stems from a theological origin. That theology also establishes the principles of the bioethical viewpoint in Catholicism. That is, created in the image and likeness of God, 'man' has an eminent dignity which allows him to share in the divine life of God. Elsewhere, the Magisterium also considers the sin of man and his redemption in Christ.

The image of God and human dignity

The Apostolic Letter of John Paul II, *Mulieris Dignitatem* (1988), on the dignity and vocation of woman, referring to the account in the Book of Genesis, states:

> [In] the setting of the biblical "beginning" ... the revealed truth concerning man as "the image and likeness" of God constitutes the immutable basis of all Christian anthropology. (6)

'Man's' dignity is at the core of the above anthropological reality, and is highlighted in the *Catechism of the Catholic Church* (1995):

> Being in the image of God the human individual possesses the dignity of a person, who is not just something, but someone. He is capable of self-knowledge, of self-possession and of freely giving himself and entering into communion with other persons. And he is called by grace to a covenant with his Creator, to offer him a response of faith and love that no other creature can give in his stead. (357)

The concept of human dignity finds its origins in God's creation of 'man' in His image and likeness, whereby every human person has the capacity to be a moral subject through the use of their intellectual rational faculty, and their free-will (Fisichella, 1993). This likeness to God is an indication that 'man' is: "the only creature on earth which God willed for itself" (*Gaudium et Spes*, Second Vatican Council 1965, 24). The theme of the *Imago Dei* (Jonsson, 1988) constantly recurs in the history of Christian anthropology and in the writing of the Fathers of the Catholic Church, whereby 'man' has a rational character, a capacity for intellectual knowledge, and possesses free will.

The theological teaching of the Catholic Church specifies Adam as being both the first man and the figure of the one who would come, Christ the Lord. This is a fundamental affirmation whereby Christ, the 'new Adam', makes 'man' known to himself in the revelation of the mystery and love of the Father. Christ also provides 'man' the possibility and the capacity to discover the magnificence of his vocation. It is not surprising then that the truths recalled above find in Him their origin and reach through Him their climax. In this regard, *Gaudium et Spes* (Second Vatican Council, 1965) states:

> He Who is "the image of the invisible God" (Col. 1:15), is Himself the perfect man. To the sons of Adam He restores the divine likeness which had been disfigured from the first sin onward. Since human nature as He assumed it was not annulled, by that very fact it has been raised up to a divine dignity in our respect too. For by His incarnation the Son of God has united Himself in some fashion with every man. He worked with human hands, He thought with a human mind, acted by human choice and loved with a human heart. Born of the Virgin Mary, He has truly been made one of us, like us in all things except sin. (22)

Christ is the perfect person for all humanity. By suffering for our sake, He did not simply lead by example, He also carved out a new path for us. Thus, 'man' can exist in His company with the benefit of "the power of the truth about man and the world that is contained in the mystery of the Incarnation and the Redemption and with the power of the love that is radiated by that truth" (Pope John Paul II 1979, 13).

It is therefore not a question of some abstract or general revelation of 'man,' but rather the revelation of a 'concrete' and 'historical' perspective on 'man' himself, given that "each man, for each one included in the mystery of the Redemption and with each one Christ has united himself for ever through this mystery" (Pope John Paul II 1979, 13). As such, Christ's message about human nature relates not only to the intellect or general human characteristics, but also to the personal and existential nature of each person. This reality is also clarified through the mystery of Christ, and through every person who chooses to 'participate' in this mystery and enter its 'plenitude' (Pope John Paul II 1979, 13). This participation ensures the vital communication between Christ and every human being, fulfilling human dignity, which is the foundation of Catholic anthropology.

As the image of God, 'man' enters an alliance with God that is fulfilled through filiation, love and communion. 'Man' as a creature experiences a conflict wherein at one point he experiences the limitations of life, but conversely also feels the calling of the superior life (Second Vatican Council 1965, 10). The dignity, value and autonomy of every person represent a characteristic element of Catholic anthropology, and thus can be considered as the main reason for the birth of a personalist approach to bioethics.

The intermediary between God and every creature is the humanity of Christ, where 'man' is the image of Jesus Christ, who is Himself the image of God the Father, and thus transcends human nature. The incarnation reveals the Christic dimension of 'man,' and that enables the human person to complete an authentic communion with God. Faggioni (1995) states that by becoming flesh, the Son of God has forever united His flesh with that of 'man.' It is worth noting that in Biblical terms, 'flesh' also connotes the frailty of 'man' as a creature, as well as Christ becoming flesh. As such, the human mode of existence is one whereby humanity is created to be fragile, ill, distressed and mortal (Faggioni, 1995).

The dignity of the human person, based on the image of God, is fundamental to Catholic bioethics. Furthermore, this dignity becomes the focus of 'normative Catholic ethics' concerning the respect due to 'man' for the simple fact that he is 'man' (Pontifical Council for Health Pastoral Care 1995, 6).

The human being is both corporeal and spiritual

The second Biblical recitation of creation presents the human person, created in the image of God, as a being that is both corporeal and spiritual. The Book of Genesis makes use of symbolic language to express this reality, stating that:

> Yahweh God shaped man from the soil of the ground and blew the breath of life into his nostrils, and man became a living being. (Gen 2:7)

'Man' is thus completely and utterly sought after by God.

Similarly, human life is decisively corporeal and spiritual (Pontifical Council for Health Pastoral Care 1995, 39), insofar as 'man' is an incarnated spirit, which means a soul expressed in a human body. The body is, in its turn, animated by an immortal spirit (Pope John Paull II, 1981). Further, it is stated that:

> By virtue of its substantial union with a spiritual soul, the human body cannot be considered as a mere complex of tissues, organs and functions ... it is a constitutive part of the person who manifests and expresses himself through it. (Congregation For The Doctrine Of The Faith 1987, 3)

Human nature then, allows the person to be fulfilled as a 'unified totality.' John Paul II (1983) also states that:

> Every human person, in its unique singularity, is not solely

constituted by the spirit, but also by the body, in a way that in the body and through the body the person himself is attained in his concrete reality.

The reality of the unified human person is also followed through in the *Catechism of the Catholic Church* (1995), stating that:

> The unity of soul and body is so profound that one has to consider the soul to be the "form" of the body: i.e., it is because of its spiritual soul that the body made of matter becomes a living, human body; spirit and matter, in man, are not two natures united, but rather their union forms a single nature. (365)

When reflecting upon the dignity of the human being, the consequences of the unity between body and soul are endless. This too, is referred to in the *Catechism of the Catholic Church* (1995):

> In Sacred Scripture the term "soul" often refers to human life or the entire human person. But "soul" also refers to the innermost aspect of man, that which is of greatest value in him, that by which he is most especially in God's image: "soul" signifies the spiritual principle in man. (363)

From the above, the vision of 'man' can now be seen to be a sacred vision. This is the contribution of Christian anthropology to bioethical discussion. Human beings are then a unity of the corporeal and spiritual, worthy of respect, and thus any intervention upon the human body must be tested by its effect upon the totality of the person. As such, Catholic bioethics perceives the inviolability of the human person in all situations and circumstances.

"Man and woman, He created them" – equal in dignity

In the Book of Genesis, the first text of human creation does not offer any differentiation between the creation of man and woman: "... male and female, He created them" (Gen 1:27). This brief yet concise statement establishes the foundation of equality between man and woman, which is the central principle of Christian anthropology. Pope John Paul II (1988) furthers this concept in the *Mulieris Dignitatem*, stating that:

> ... man is the highpoint of the whole order of creation in the visible world; the human race, which takes its origin from the calling into existence of man and woman, crowns the whole work of creation; both man and woman are human beings to an equal degree, both are created in God's image. (6)

The second text about human creation in the Book of Genesis does not, in essence, contradict the first. However, the language used bears a different connotation when describing the creation of woman. In fact, woman was created by God from the rib of man (Gen 2:18-25). In *Mulieris Dignitatem* (1988), Pope John Paul II interprets the creation of woman as:

> ... another "I" in a common humanity. From the very beginning they appear as a "unity of the two", and this signifies that the original solitude is overcome, the solitude in which man does not find "a helper fit for him" (Gen 2:20). (6)

Additionally, the Biblical term *ishsha*, implies that the identity of the woman is formed concurrently with the identity of man, *ish*. This then asserts that woman is "a being equal to man in nature and dignity" (Haring 1989, p. 595).

These two texts from the Book of Genesis provide a base that acknowledges the essential equality between man and woman in humanity. This is supported by the Fathers of the Church – in particular Origen, Clement of Alexandria and Augustine – who affirmed the fundamental equality between man and woman before God. Both man and woman were created by God and therefore both wanted by God:

> Man and woman have been created, which is to say, willed by

God: on the one hand, in perfect equality as human persons; on the other, in their respective beings as man and woman. "Being man" or "being woman" is a reality which is good and willed by God: man and woman possess an inalienable dignity which comes to them immediately from God their Creator. (Catechism of the Catholic Church 1995, 369)

Man and woman are equal in dignity, because they were created "in the image of God."

Pope John Paul II (1985) stated that the "perfections" of man and woman are the partial reflection of the infinite perfection of God. In being man and in being woman, which means sexual beings, man and woman are the expression of the wisdom and goodness of their Creator, in terms of their equality and physical differences, as intended by God. Additionally, the reference to 'human being' as a person led Pope John Paul II (1988) to conclude that 'man' is a person regardless of their sexual being.

In Catholic bioethics, there is no justification for sexual discrimination. The human person is respected for who they are, and not for their gender. The core of this respect is the anthropological principle of equality in dignity between man and woman.

'Man' and the universe: the shared lordship or "seigniority"

Even though the Book of Genesis does not explain the nature of 'man' being in the resemblance of God, it does highlight the purpose of 'man's' creation in the image of God. 'Man' is called to be the master and protector of life, following God the Creator who loved His creation. The Magisterium also puts forward the notion of the human being as a participant in the lordship or 'seigniory' of God, to ensure loyalty towards God's aim in the creation (Faggioni, 1995).

The Biblical view of existence can only be understood through the relationship between God and the creation. That is, God is the sole Lord, and the ultimate reference for all existence, present, past and future. Therefore, in the creation God ordered 'man' to "fill the earth and subdue it" (Gen 1:28). This means that man has a position of superiority over the universe (John Paul II, 1985).

'Man' exerts a domination that does not oppose, but presupposes and proposes the supreme domination of God. The encyclical letter of Pope John Paul II, *Evangelium Vitae* (1995) explains the original nature of the lordship as:

> To defend and promote life, to show reverence and love for it, is a task which God entrusts to every man, calling him as his living image to share in his own lordship over the world. (42)

'Man' then is in a position that permits the exercising of authentic lordship over non-human life, and is consequently in a position of responsibility for all living nature.

Given that 'man's' lordship is shared, 'man' is then not in a position to take an authoritarian stance or destroy the intrinsic dynamics of God's creation. Every being in God's creation has the right to exist as God intended.

If 'man' is the lord of all creatures he must not forget that 'he' is one of them. As such, Faggioni (1995) describes humanity as being:

> ... one of the creatures, but of all the created are laid by God at the feet of man, or to bemore precise, under (Hebrew: tahat) the feet of man ... This superior dignity of man justifies the domination of man over the created things. (pp. 430-431)

Further to the above, the encyclical letter of Pope John Paul II *Centesimus Annus* (1991) suggests that the modern ecological and environmental crises being experienced are due to the errors of humankind, where humanity:

> ... forgets that this is ... God's prior and original gift...[and] thinks that he can make arbitrary use of the earth...which man can indeed develop but must not betray. (37)

After confirming 'man's' lordship and limits, *Evangelium Vitae* (Pope John Paul II, 1995) elaborates the most significant aspect of the shared lordship: lordship over human life. The participation of 'man' in God's lordship becomes more obvious in the responsibility entrusted to man and woman regarding human life. This responsibility will culminate when man and woman in marriage realise that:

> ... the task of accepting and serving life involves everyone; and this task must be fulfilled above all towards life when it is at its weakest. (43)

Catholic bioethics explains that the right of 'man' to be in command of any intervention upon his own physical being is consistent with the theological view of the Church. This balanced position highlights the fact that 'man' having real lordship over creatures and his own life, must not take advantage and abuse life. 'Man' must follow the divine model of lordship, exercising lordship with wisdom and love:

> For man, created to God's image, received a mandate to subject to himself the earth and all it contains, and to govern the world with justice and holiness; a mandate to relate himself and the totality of things to Him Who was to be acknowledged as the Lord and Creator of all. Thus, by the subjection of all things to man, the name of God would be wonderful in all the earth. (Second Vatican Council 1965, 34)

The *Catechism of the Catholic Church* (1995) reasserts the position expressed in various Magisteriums, in that the shared lordship of 'man' is based on love, and:

> In God's plan man and woman have the vocation of "subduing" the earth (Gen 1:28) as stewards of God. This sovereignty is not to be an arbitrary and destructive domination. God calls man and woman, made in the image of the Creator "who loves everything that exists" (Wis 11:24), to share in his providence toward other creatures;

hence their responsibility for the world God has entrusted to them. (373)

The Second Vatican Council in *Gaudium et Spes* (1965) supports this by referring to the Book of Sirach (Sr 15:14) which states that God enabled 'man' to search for his creator "subject to their own decisions" (17). 'Man' will freely reach Him, and in doing so 'man' will reach happiness. Accordingly, *Veritatis Splendor* (Pope John Paul II, 1993) refers to:

> ... the wonderful depth of the sharing in God's dominion to which man has been called: they indicate that man's dominion extends in a certain sense over man himself ... Thus human nature, created to rule other creatures, was by its likeness to the King of the universe made as it were a living image, partaking with the Archetype both in dignity and in name. (38)

The vocation of man: to be with God

According to Christian anthropology, 'man' cannot be thought of without a profound relationship with God. The vocation of 'man' originates in his resemblance to God, which places him in a live relationship with creative love. *Evangelium Vitae* implies that 'man' is:

> ... called to a fullness of life which far exceeds the dimensions of his earthly existence, because it consists in sharing the very life of God. (Pope John Paul II 1995, 2)

This supernatural vocation as expressed in *Evangelium Vitae* (Pope John Paul II 1995, 2) reveals the magnificence and worth of human life in its temporal phase. In fact, the earthly life of man and woman is not a *final reality* but a *before-final reality*. In all cases, it is a *sacred reality*, whereby:

> ... having been created in the image of God ... all men are called to one and the same goal, namely God Himself. (Second Vatican Council 1965, 24)

Only 'man' is created in the image of God alone. Therefore, he cannot long for or exist for any other, but only God. As such, the vocation of 'man' must be at the level of a relationship of love with the Creator. The *Catechism of the Catholic Church* (1995) emphasises this:

> Of all visible creatures only man is "able to know and love his creator." He is "the only creature on earth that God has willed for its own sake", and he alone is called to share, by knowledge and love, in God's own life. (356)

The history of the relationship between 'man' and his Creator has had to endure hard challenges. After receiving the spirit of life from God, Adam had become a living human being. To the breathed spirit of life, God added His Word, and this first word took the form of a prohibition:

> Then Yahweh God gave the man this command, 'You are free to eat of all the tress in the garden. But of the tree of the knowledge of good and evil you are not to eat; for, the day you eat of that, you are doomed to die.' (Gen 2:16-17)

'Man' is united to his Creator through a dependant and vital relationship where his freedom must be expressed under the form of obedience. Yet, *Veritatis Splendor* (Pope John Paul II, 1993) states that:

> God's law does not reduce, much less do away with human freedom; rather, it protects and promotes that freedom. (35)

However, Adam disobeyed God and "ate from the tree."

Adam's disobedience in effect ruptured his relationship with the source of life, and as a consequence of this sin, death entered into the world. The first couple wanted to eat the fruit of the tree in order to become like God. Pope John Paul II (1988) explains that, in this sinful act 'man' rejected God's gift of supernatural happiness which arises from 'man's' participation in God's life. That is:

> Sin brings about a break in the original unity which man enjoyed in the state of original justice: union with God as the source of the unity within his own "I", in the mutual relationship between man and woman ("communio personarum") as well as in regard to the external world, to nature. (9)

Before announcing the change that will affect 'man,' God plants the hope of redemption in his heart (Gen 3:15). The sinner, Adam, cannot return to what was – *in the image of God* – but he will be reshaped *in the image of Christ*: not simply in the image of the Word, but in the image of the Crucified, victorious over sin and death (Pope John Paul II 1979, 8). Adam can only find the meaning of his being and his existence within Jesus Christ, the Son of God who was made man for all to become children of God (Gal 4:4-5). The new covenant welcomes humanity in the unity of the *Person of the Word* who reconciles 'man' with his Creator (Pope John Paul II 1988, 9). Christ, and after Him, all the believers, represent the new 'man.' With Him, 'man' is no longer a simple mortal, for faith has planted in his heart the seed of immortality. The old 'man' must incessantly die in order to be reborn, new, through Jesus Christ (2 Co 3:18); thus, man "...is renewed in the image of its Creator" (Col 3: 10) by action of the Holy Spirit (*Gaudium et Spes,* Second Vatican Council 1965, 13 and 22).

God wants to bring all men to a life of communion with Him. In the Old Testament, the theme of the covenant, dominated by this idea, is fundamental to Biblical religious thought. However, it only reaches its climax in the New Testament, namely through Jesus Christ, because "Christ is in a way united with every man, even when man is unaware of it." (Pope John Paul II 1979, 14). That is, Christ is united with every man through the new covenant which he established between God and humanity.

The sanctity of human life is the fundamental principle of Catholic bioethics, where:

> Human life is sacred because from its beginning it involves "the creative action of God" and it remains forever in a special relationship with the Creator, who is its sole end. (Congregation For The Doctrine Of The Faith 1987, 5)

Among the numerous biblical references which profess this reality, the inspiring words of Psalm 139 highlight it, stating:

> You created my inmost self,
> knit me in my mother's womb ...
> You knew me through and through,
> my being held no secrets from you.
> when I was being formed in secret,
> textured in the depths of the earth.
> Your eyes could see my embryo.
> In your book all my days were inscribed,
> everyone that was fixed is there.

The value of human life is not the result of any subject's actions or words , but rather resides in the fact of existence and being in a relationship with God. The value of the inviolability of human life finds its roots *per ultimo* in God. Young or adult, healthy or sick, embryo or new-born, genius or idiot, the value of each human being is completely independent from the quality of life. What eventually matters, is "the being in a relationship with God," so that:

> If each relationship with another is revealing my being as a person, then only the relationship with God constitutes my being person, because my being and my value do not exist outside of this relationship with the absolute and founder otherness, in a word, with God. (Faggioni 1995, p. 51)

In Summary

Based on Biblical anthropology, Christian anthropology positions 'man' as the centre of God's creative work. In Catholicism, the doctrine of the creation of humanity definitively culminates in 'man,' created in the image of God, redeemed and atoned by Jesus Christ. It is in this context that *Evangelium Vitae* (Pope John Paul II, 1995) speaks of "the incomparable value of every human person" (2). In the Magisterium, 'man' is an incarnate spirit situated in space and time. Even though 'man' does experience a certain tension between these two dimensions of his being, he always subsists as a substantial union between the body and the spirit, in every action and decision made. From this he derives his specific *unitotality*. Furthermore, man and woman, both being created in the image and likeness of God, are equal in nature and dignity. However, equality and dignity will only prosper through a bond and unity with God.

It can be argued then, that as 'man' is one of God's creatures, he is inconceivable outside of a relationship with his Creator. The relationship that exists between each human being and their Creator is absolutely unique. It is also a personal, constitutive and exclusive relationship, where 'man' becomes a person, a universal self-transcendent reality, and in the All, open to others in their 'otherness.' Ingrained in the Sacred Scriptures, the vocation of 'man' is thus a vital connection to God, through Jesus Christ. It is this concept of 'man' that allows us to maintain that Catholic bioethics, by its *personalist* character, draws its foundations and principles from Christian anthropology.

Finally, God's evaluation of His creation reaches its completion as a whole which is intrinsically good (Pope John Paul II 1985), that is, "God saw all he had made, and indeed it was very good" (Gen 1:31).

2

Bioethics and the Concept of Man in Islam

The concept of man in Islam is essentially based on the Koranic text, and as such allows for an exclusively Koranic anthropology. The difference between Catholicism and Islam is that Christian anthropology is based on the Bible but has been developed, creating its own distinctive anthropology, whilst Islamic anthropology is confined and limited to the Koran.

Islam reminds man that everything is given to him through Allah. Therefore, man must not forget this fundamental truth that "nothing that exists is explained without Allah." In this context, Islamic bioethics is situated in direct connection with the *Shari'a*, so that its teachings are legalist rather than anthropological. As such, the following discussion will primarily focus on the Koranic text to explain the Islamic concept of the creation of man and woman. The *Shari'a* will also be referred to, further on in the discussion.

Creation of man in the Islamic theological tradition

In its text about the creation, the Koran positions man as a servant and worshiper of Allah. Man was created to be a gifted worshiper with the ability to receive Allah's Revelation, and to believe in both Allah and His prophet. Furthermore, if man is required to lead the perfect Muslim life, he will receive the rewards outlined by the Koran, in the future life. Man in Islam, is thus a privileged being who was made by the hands of the Creator, as viceroy of the universe (Masson, 1976).

The creation of man according to the Koran
Derived from Biblical anthropology, the Koran presents a lengthy

reflection on Allah the Creator and on the first created man (Borrmans, 1993), as evidenced through the numerous Koranic verses that refer to the creation and to the origin of man. However, before discussing the creation of man and woman, it is important to note two concepts that are featured in the Koran – the creation of man through *separation*, and *Koranic embryogenesis* which is the creation of man in *successive phases*.

Translators of the Koran have rendered the verb *fatara* as *'create'*. But the proper Arabic word for 'create' is *'khalaqa'*. It is important to note that this process of coming into being occurred *by a kind of separation*, and was from something that already existed. This separation, which is the origin of man, expressed by the verb *fatara*, confirms the specific differentiation of human nature known in the Koran as the *fitra*, a derivative of *fatara* (Talbi and Bucaille, 1989). The verb *fatara* is linked to the creation or apparition of man, and is found in five different Koranic verses, one of which states:

> O my people! I ask of you no reward for it. Lo! My reward is the concern only of Him who made me [*fatarani*]. Have ye then no sense? (11:51)

In the four further verses 20:72, 43:27, 36:22 and 17:51, and the one quoted above, Allah presents Himself as the One who created man *by separation*. This concept is defined by Jomier (1996) who ascertains that *fitra* refers to *nature* as created by Allah, holding His imprint and oriented towards Him. Jomier adds that the chosen meaning for *fatara* is "nature seen through the eyes of a man of faith", and also points out the meaning of *fitra* in Arabic dictionaries being either 'creation' or 'separation and rupture' (1996, p. 35).

The other form of creation referred to in the Koran is through *successive phases*:

> What aileth you that ye hope not toward Allah for dignity
> When He created you by (divers) stages? (71:13-14)

Creation through successive phases is expounded in various verses in the Koran, which describe the various phases, for example:

> Verily We created man from a product of wet earth;
>
> Then placed him as a drop (of seed) in a safe lodging;
>
> Then fashioned We the drop a clot, then fashioned We the clot a little lump, then fashioned We the little lump bones, then clothed the bones with flesh, and then produced it as another creation. So blessed be Allah, the Best of Creators! (23:12-14)

Talbi and Bucaille (1989) present the different forms of clay Allah used to create man: *"from a product of wet earth"* (23: 12), or *"plastic clay"* (37:11), or *"clay like the potter's"* (55: 14) or finally *"potter's clay of black mud"* (15:26 and 15:28). Al-Bar (1995) adds that the creation in successive *phases* may be interpreted in a chronological and spatial manner in reference to the different stages of growth of the fetus "in three veils of darkness" in the mother's womb, and is stated in the Koran thus: "He created you in the wombs of your mothers, creation after creation, in a threefold gloom" (39:6).

Evidently, the created being has progressed through various stages of growth and is an evolved matter of the earth. The creation through *successive phases* illustrates that Adam was not the child of a couple, but a parcel of life made from the earth a long time ago and born according to the order of *the most skilful* creator. As such, the creation of man in *successive phases* began as *clay* which is a matter *prepared* to give life. What does this mean? Talbi and Bucaille (1989) assert that the matter itself goes through numerous phases or *atwar*, before becoming adequately prepared to give birth to the first living element. Clearly, man is not a pottery. Nonetheless, he is an evolved matter that stems from the earth. Before being the child of a couple, born from the union of an ovum and a spermatozoon, Adam was for a long time a mere parcel of life directly conceived in the womb of the earth. Allah who has created everything by destiny *(qadar)* is the Almighty Architect who has programmed and directed everything towards a distant target, that is, man.

As previously mentioned, the mode of creation is a *separation* by *successive phases*. This was the means of preparing the appearance of the first human being on earth. The Koran considers Adam to be the first man. The word 'Adam' has the same meaning as in the Bible. It is a reference to the surface of the ground. The word, in its Arabic as well as its Hebrew form, is a derivative of a proto-Semitic root. According to the Koran, the first man was created from *dust (turāb)* (3:59; 30:20; 40:67) or *clay (tīn)* (6:2; 32:7).

Seven verses of the Koran describe how Allah created Adam, one of which states that:

> And when thy Lord said unto the angels: Lo! I am about to place a viceroy in the earth, they said: wilt Thou place therein one who will do harm therein and will shed blood, while we, we hymn Thy praise and sanctify Thee? He said: Surely I know that which ye know not.
>
> And He taught Adam all the names, then showed them to the angels, saying: Inform me of the names of these, if ye are truthful.
>
> They said: Be glorified! We have no knowledge saving that which Thou hast taught us. Lo! Thou, only Thou, art the Knower, the Wise.
>
> He said: O Adam! Inform them of their names, and when he had informed them of their names, He said: Did I not tell you that I know the secret of the heavens and the earth? And I know that which ye disclose and which ye hide.
>
> And when We said unto the angels: Prostrate yourselves before Adam, they fell prostrate, all save Iblis. He demurred through pride, and so became a disbeliever. (2:30-34)

Using more or less identical terms, and in more or less a concise manner, the Koran elsewhere recounts the history of the creation of man by Allah (Abbud 1978; Fahd 1959; Arnaldez 1971). It is noted that:

1. The Koran contains seven references to the creation of man. Six are from the Mecca period, and one from the Medina period.
2. Allah was not alone. The Angels and particularly Iblis, who had a particular status among them, also existed.
3. The sky was not empty, and a large creation was already in existence.
4. Harmony reigned and evil was excluded. The Angels glorified Allah and proclaimed His holiness.
5. In this harmony, Iblis, the enigmatic being whose name is derived from the Greek word *diabolos*, had the doubtful ability to either obey or disobey.

With reference to the primary matter of which man was created, the Koran mentions dust and fine clay. The following two verses confirm an aquatic version of the origin of life:

> Allah hath created every animal of water. (24:45)
>
> and
>
> And He it is Who hath created man from water ... (25:54)

It appears from the above that man was created from water, as were all other living beings. Clay and spirit are not mentioned in this context.

Koranic anthropology confers a great value on man, whom Allah created with soil and clay (Al-Naggar 1996; Arnaldez 1971), and then harmoniously formed, blowing His spirit into him, and bestowing him with a body and a soul. Allah placed man above the heavens, earth and the angels, who must prostrate themselves before Him, and then made man master of the angels by teaching him the names of all things, which in Semitic tradition means to know and dominate them (Borrmans, 1993). Significantly, Allah made man his vicar on earth (2:28), which in Islamic doctrine means that the honour and greatness of Islamic man results from the privileges bestowed on him by Allah, and by carrying out His orders and sanctions. The secret of Allah's choice of man can only be understood through the initial *mithaq* or pact between the Creator and His creation.

The word *mithaq* is not accurately translated as 'pact' or 'alliance'. The literal meaning of the word is 'a solid bond', or 'a reliable, trustworthy engagement'. In contrast, Jewish-Christian theological terminology refers to an essential concept of the "economy of salvation" which is based on the "chronological" election of the people of Israel and, which later on spread to include all those redeemed by Christ's sacrifice on the cross. Evidently, this depiction is entirely foreign to the spirit of the Koran. (Talbi and Bucaille, 1989).

However, Koranic man, who is presented with honour and greatness, is at the same time a faithful servant of his Lord, and, ontologically speaking, a weak and perishable creature. To further emphasise the nature of man, Allah in the Koran repeatedly reminds him of his condition as a frail and weak creature. (Abd Al-Rahman, 1978). Man is simply soil and clay, and is unfair and confused (33:70), and being ungrateful, he contributes to his own downfall (113:2 and 22:65). Man also displays his ungrateful nature to his Lord, as noted in the Koran (100:6). Additionally, man is rebellious (96:6), a liar with criminal traits (96:16), miserable, impatient, and unreliable (70:18-19); and everything is controversial through his eyes (18:52).

The creation of woman according to the Koran

The creation of the first woman deserves particular attention because Allah, according to the Koran, states:

> ... He created for you helpmeets from yourselves that ye might find rest in them ... (30:21)

The Koranic affirmation that woman was created from man, reflects the Biblical verse about the creation of woman (Gen 2:21-22). However, the Koran does not specify the way in which Allah created woman, and presents the woman as man's wife:

> And We said: O Adam! Dwell thou and thy wife in the Garden, and eat ye freely (of the fruits) thereof where ye will; but come not nigh this tree lest ye become wrongdoers. (2:35)

From the above verse, Allah speaks simultaneously and equally to Adam and his wife, who has not been named. This sin is made through a sanction: do not touch the Tree of Life. Both Adam and his wife were implicated in their choice that is based on the human freedom of determination (Abd Al-Rahman, 1978).

Man according to the contemporary Shari'a

A clear Koranic concept of man emerges from the numerous verses that narrate the creation, whereby one perspective presents greatness and superiority, and another presents misery and slavery encountered in human life. The *Shari'a* takes these concepts and attempts to apply them to the daily life of the Muslim man. Allah, in the *Shari'a*, makes Himself known to Adam through Eve when He created man and woman, and all that exists. Like the Biblical story of Adam and Eve in paradise, the Koran makes reference to Adam's sin and repentance. Allah punishes Adam, who by disobeying had become sinful. But Allah forgives Adam and his wife when Adam repents, and so Allah promises to guide them with His mercy (20:123-124). Unlike Judaism and Christianity, Islam maintains that it was the first man Adam who committed the sin, and not his wife. The *Shari'a* explains how Adam forgot and disobeyed his Lord, and then his woman disobeyed following his lead (Abdel-Wahab, 1994).

The concept of man and women according to the *Shari'a*, is simply a development of Koranic anthropology. Man is Allah's vicar on earth, bound to his Creator by a pact (*mithaq*) and by the weight of Allah's *amana* or trust in man, who is both body and soul.

Unlike the thought of the Catholic Church, woman is not equal to man, given her dependence on man.

It is also worth noting the beneficial lordship of man over the universe, where man is allowed to take advantage of his superiority over all other living creatures. His vocation is to serve and worship Allah.

Man is the successor (khalifa) of God in the universe, the vicarial mission, and the dignity

The *Shari'a* presents two key roles for man, a vicarial mission and a responsibility assumed through the pact *(mithaq)*. This pact *(mithaq)* between Allah and man is realised through the revelation of a natural religion *(fitra)*, in which man is valued by his desire to preserve the trust *(amana)* given to him.

The vicarial mission of man taught in the *Shari'a*, is based on the following Koranic verse:

> And when thy Lord said unto the angels: Lo! I am about to place a viceroy in the earth, they said: Wilt Thou place therein one who will do harm therein and will shed blood, while we, we hymn Thy praise and sanctify Thee? He said: Surely I know that which ye know not. (2:30)

From the above verse, some aspects of man's vicarial mission emerge:

1. The creation of Adam relates to his planned mission, namely, that he has been chosen by Allah to be His representative, His vicar-successor or *khalifa* on earth (Abd Al-Rahman, 1978). However, most commentators and orientalists draw on certain Koranic verses, where man is identified as *khalifa*, to infer that he is the vicar *of God* on earth, his lieutenant and his representative among other

creatures. Accordingly, this warrants the dominion that he can and must exercise on these creatures. Nevertheless, the use of the word *khalifa* in the Koran leaves no room for such an interpretation. The verb *khalafa* means "to succeed somebody" or "to inherit something". The only possible translation in compatibility with the context of these verses is "successor" or "heir". However, the Koran offers no reason for the proposition that man is the successor or the heir *of God* on earth. Moreover, this claim goes against Koranic theology that asserts that no one can replace or represent Allah. This vicarial mission entrusted to man is the reason why his life on earth is directed towards doing good and avoiding evil and that he must take full responsibility for his actions as well as the choices he makes.

2. The choice of Allah to favour man was unexpected by the angels, who were Allah's "obedient servants," yet expressed spite and jealousy when He favoured "one who will do harm therein and will shed blood, while we, we hymn Thy praise and sanctify Thee."

3. Allah's response, "Surely I know that which ye know not," shows His omniscience as well as the angels' "limited" knowledge.

4. To confirm man's superiority over the angels, Allah "taught Adam all the names" (2:31), thus making man responsible for teaching the angels (2:31).

5. The handing over of the earth to man reveals his vicarial mission.

Man is only able to fully practise his vicariate if he is loyal to his primary vocation, which is to be a witness and worshiper of the unique Allah, as "Unto Allah belongeth the Sovereignty of the heavens and the earth" (3:189). In the same way, Gardet (1967, p. 51) quotes one Hadith which states that "the earth belongs to Allah and the Muslims."

Therefore man does not have the right to *use or abuse* his power. Allah possess the supreme authority *(mulk)* over all things, which are at his disposal. Accordingly, Allah will bless the loyal man with earthly rewards, and punish the impious.

In this regard, Jomier (1996) states that the vicarial mission is one of the principal components of the dignity of man according to the *Shari'a* of Allah. Other verses also evoke, more or less clearly, the dignity of man (2:31-33).

Man is chosen by Allah to assume the vicariate role, although Allah's expectations must be fulfilled and His sanctions must be respected. This then, implies the "election of the human race", for:

> Verily We have honoured the children of Adam. We carry them on the land and the sea, and have made provision of good things for them, and have preferred them above many of those whom We created with a marked preferment. (17:70)

Allah has bequeathed man with a free will, to enable him to manage as he wishes the expectations and sanctions that man must obey. According to Islamic theology, Allah imposes law over man. He rewards for obedience and punishes in the case of transgressions. However, the Koran remains ambiguous on the matter of free will, including both verses supporting freedom and others which stand in opposition to it (Brague, 1998).

Two additional components of the vicarial mission of man relate to the pact *(mithaq)* between Allah and man, and the "reward given by Allah to man who has accepted to bear the trust *(amana)*." This leads to a simpler understanding of Adam as the "father of human kind," whose dignity and honour are reflected in his vicariate (Abd Al-Rahman, 1978).

The Koran states:

> And (remember) when they Lord brought forth from the Children of Adam, from their reins, their seed, and made

> them testify of themselves, (saying): Am I not your Lord? They said: Yea, verily. We testify. (That was) lest ye should say at the Day of Resurrection: Lo! of this we were unaware. (7:172)

The pact *(mithaq)* referred to in the above verse was an initial pact, a solemn and pre-eternal engagement that has been directly sealed and defined in ontological timelessness of Allah acting "without the chronological mediation or otherwise, the intervention of a chosen people or redeeming sacrifice" (Talbi and Bucaille 1989, p.108). As a result, no man is omitted from the pact *(mithaq)* in Islam. This election, whether it concerns an individual or a group, is earned, gained or lost. All will be judged on their faithfulness to the pre-existential pact *(mithaq)*, which stamps the faith in their hearts. The pact *(mithaq)* can then be regarded as a core concept in Islamic theology.

Due to the pact *(mithaq)*, also known as the pre-existential testimony *(shahadat al-dahr,)* every man as a free ego in a decisive face-to-face with Allah, has responded to the question "Am I not your Lord?" with a "Yes" of testimony and engagement. Then, the pact *(mithaq)* naturally, directly and individually unites all Muslims, including all men, past, present and future, who positively answer the Koranic call.

Bound by the pact *(mithaq)* and enlightened by Allah's spirit *(ruh)*, Muslim man is viewed in an intimate relationship with Allah who trusts him with the *amana* (Talbi and Bucaille, 1989). Interpreting the meaning of trust *(amana)*, Talbi and Bucaille (1989) claim that this trust *(amana)* is presented as a precious trust. The trust is unique and can only be entrusted to the loyal faithful *(amin)*. In fact, it involves a hazard, it requires responsible, free and willing adherence from the receiver, in addition to loyalty and fidelity. As the trust *(amana)* is a supreme responsibility and a mutual *act of faith*, the Koran states:

> Lo! We offered the trust unto the heavens and the earth and the hills, but they shrank from bearing it and were afraid of

it. And man assumed it. Lo! he hath proved a tyrant and a fool. (33:72)

In this unique verse where man accepts the trust *(amana)* that was offered *(arada)* by Allah to the heavens, the earth and the mountains, who rejected the trust *(amana)* with horror and fear. It is to be noted that the term used is 'offered' *(arada)*, not 'imposed'. Man, who was seen as frail, was not solicited, but spontaneously accepted. Man, who accepted the trust *(amana)* was described at the end of the above verse, as a "tyrant" *(zalum)* and a "fool" *(gahul)*. The first term is derived from a word that bears a connotation of darkness as well as disorder and injustice, *zulm*; while the second term is derived from *gahl* which signifies ignorance, rudeness, irascibility, violence and brutality (Talbi and Bucaille, 1989).

The content of the trust *(amana)* seems to indicate a "Clef-de-Voute" or keystone in the order of the creation, that is a 'decisive and magnificent mission' which also carries danger and risk, and which is something to be afraid of. Overestimating himself, man, with enthusiasm and courage, freely accepts the challenge. However, the Koran does not reveal, either directly or indirectly, the aim, nature or content of the trust *(amana)* (Talbi and Bucaille, 1989).

The trust *(amana)* as it appears in the Koran is without doubt the most ambiguous and mysterious mission entrusted to man (Abd Al-Rahman, 1978). Thus the trust *(amana)*:

> ... bears different meanings, the interpreters (*'ulama'*) have yet to reach a consensus over its significance. (Al-Naggar 1996, p. 26)

Nonetheless, man is put forth as the executor of a "project" regarded as magnificent and perilous, but for which neither the heavens nor the earth nor the mountains would take responsibility.

Islamic bioethics explores the above noted facts regarding man, so as to provide an anthropological foundation to its directives and views.

Man is body and spirit

It is apparent that man in Islam is the union of body and spirit with the breath *(ruh)* of Allah, is engaged in the pact *(mithaq)* and is a recipient of trust *(amana)*. Man is forever bound to Allah by his indestructible transcendental commitment to testimony and loyalty. The Islamic doctrine regarding man as the union of body and soul originates from verse 38:72-73 in the Koran which states:

> When thy Lord said unto the angels: lo! I am about to create a mortal out of mire,
>
> And when I have fashioned him and breathed into him My spirit, then fall down before him prostrate.

The Islamic scholar Razi, as referenced by Aqqad (1973), supports the Koranic view of man, stating that he is an essence composed of a soul and a body. He asserts that the human person is the union of corporeal and spiritual being, whilst also accepting the view of Greek philosophy which examines the conflict between the body and the soul. That is, the body is attached to the earth and its 'animal' instincts and passions, whereas the spirit is elevated towards heaven. Yet, it is important to find that balance which can satisfy both facets of the human person (Aqqad, 1973). Moreover Aqqad (1973) highlights that the breath *(ruh)* received by man is not the human soul, but in this context, the source of life.

Further to the above, Al-Qaradhawi (1973) asserts:

> Islamic doctrine does not fail to acknowledge that the spirit was intended for the body and the body for the spirit, but it reunites the pair in a harmonious and complete unity, whilst giving the spirit and the body each its right, without abuse or exaggeration. (pp. 76-77)

The concept of the Muslim man can be further defined as a weak and perishable being made from clay and soil, into whom Allah has breathed His spirit, and having done so, asks a question and makes a declaration:

> Who created thee, then fashioned, then proportioned thee?
> Into whatsoever form He will, He casteth thee. (82:7-8)

In this way, from one perspective, Koranic man appears in his grandeur, while from another, he appears in his misery. Al-Buti (1992) bases himself on both perspectives to speak of a Koranic anthropology, and concludes that man, a frail being created from soil, is a slave of Allah. However, after receiving the trust *(amana)*, he becomes worthy of eminence and power. These two facts are the principle of man's Koranic education. Furthermore, this grandeur is because he is anchored in Allah, carrying within him something divine – the spirit of Allah (Talbi and Bucaille, 1989). As Allah's vicar, he was created to adore and obey Him and to work to maintain the earth. Al-Naggar (1996) offers an explanation, pointing out that the adoration of Allah is not to satisfy a divine need to be adored or praised, nor is it an expression of divine perfection. The adoration of Allah is, rather, the purpose of creation; being a slave is a benefit for the worshiper. The misery of Koranic man comes about because he is merely a being made of "mud and blood" (Al-Buti, 1992) destined to perish at a time determined by Allah.

Speaking of man's death, the Koran clearly distinguishes between the spirit and the body when it refers to the exhalation of souls *(anfus)* (9:85). The Koran aims to provide a justification for the conflict between good and bad inclinations within man, which is detectable within Adam, in the conflict between his flesh of the earth and his spirit that emanates from Allah (15:29; 38:72).

The concept of physical and spiritual unity of the human person is, in general, adopted by Islam, and constitutes the basis of respecting and protecting human life. If "the body is prior and a pre-requisite to the emergence of the spirit" (Chebel 1987, p. 205), then Islamic bioethics forbids any offence against human life from the moment that it has been created when Allah sends the human soul to animate the body.

Creation of man and woman: a question of equality

To a certain degree, within Islamic thought, there is the "sacralisation" of the inferiority of woman (Tomiche, 1971). The Koran asserts that the souls of the first women or wives were stemmed from the soul of Adam: "He created for you helpmeets from yourselves" (30:21). Therefore woman is ontologically dependant on man. She is a second grade human being to be placed in the background, as she is subordinated to the male in the hierarchy of Allah's creatures, is required to fulfil certain roles and duties, and has limited power over her own future and her own body (Abbud, 1978; Yaljin 1973). Further evidence is found in the Koran of male superiority over female (2:228) such as, the requirement to have two female witnesses where one male would normally suffice (2:282); women are entitled to half the inheritance amount that men would receive (4:11-12); polygamy is authorised (4:3), as is repudiation, which is a right uniquely reserved for man (2:226-32; 66).

Thus in Muslim hierarchy, the woman is ranked alongside children, and weaker beings that require protection (7:127 and 141; 14:6; 40:25). On these principles, woman will always be held in a subordinate position by Koranic "paternalism" (Jomier, 1996; Fahd, 1959). With that in mind, equality between man and woman in Islam remains inconceivable and even impossible. Therefore, a personalist bioethical approach seems to be particularly impossible in the Islamic world.

Man and the universe – the beneficial lordship

The universe is regarded as the "scene of human action," in the *Shari'a*. It is neither the result of chance nor vanity, because the "God of ants and stars" has a determined purpose for the universe (Al-

Naggar, 1996). Furthermore, the Koran proclaims that the creation of the cosmos, that is heaven and earth, preceded the creation of man, highlighting the privileged position of man in the universe (Al-Buti, 1992). As such, the *Shari'a* defines the relationship between man and the universe through two fundamental aspects – the unity of man and the universe, and the superiority of the former over the latter.

The above distinction between man and the universe confirms the duality of their existence. However, the submission of man and the universe to Allah establishes between them a relation of unity which "the Koran and the Hadith constantly relay" (Al-Naggar 1996, p. 60). However, it is acknowledged that being created by and submitted to Allah does not always lead to the same destiny. In fact, the Koran emphasises that the elements of the universe will perish after their visible existence, whereas man, endowed with an immortal soul, will enter another life and:

> Everything will perish save His countenance. His is the command, and unto Him ye will be brought back. (28:88)

From the first verses in which Allah reveals himself to Muhammad, Allah grants man privileges:

> Read: In the name of thy Lord who createth,
> Createth man from a clot. (96:1-2)

Accordingly, "man became the centre of existence and the value of creatures is determined through their relation with him" (Al-Naggar 1996, p. 70). Man is thus distinguished from the universe by his superiority and his sublimity, as is acknowledged in the Koran:

> Verily We have honoured the children of Adam. We carry them on the land and the sea, and have made provision of good things for them, and have preferred them above many of those whom We created with a marked preferment. (17:70)

Man's superiority is also evidenced through the unification in him of the two distinct elements in the universe: the material and spiritual, with man as the unique being to encompass both (Al-Naggar 1996, p. 71). The unification of body and spirit, which is unique to man, establishes him as competent to take on the responsibility (*taklif*) and to bear the trust (*amana*), the signs of his superiority and his sublimity" (Talbi and Bucaille 1989, p. 73).

The union between man and the universe, along with the superiority of man over the universe, leads to another reality: the submission of the universe to man. Al-Naggar (1996) discusses this submission as found in the *Shari'a*, when looking at the relationship between man and the universe, stating that:

> The universe as a whole is subjugated to man, and man must subdue it, invest it and make a profit from it." (p. 76)

The universe then, was created according to fixed measures, rules and regulations, and is far from any imperfection. In brief, it has been created by Allah and submitted to man. This submission is not an end in itself, but rather arises from the divine will of Allah to give man control over the universe created before him. The submission of the universe to man in Islam raises a controversial matter: a relationship based on profit makes the emergence of ecological bioethics difficult, that is, the correlation between Islamic bioethics and environmental concerns become problematic.

In spite of his place within and relationship with the universe, Muslim man is convinced of his superiority and right to govern the universe, and as Al-Naggar (1996) states:

> Believing that the universe is subjugated to him, exclusively arranged for his existence and introduced in order for him to work and act, man thus finds himself in the centre of the interaction and harmony with the universe. (p. 97)

To illustrate the mind-set of *beneficial lordship* and explain the absence of the meaning of sacrifice in Islam, a *Hadith* quoted by Al-Naggar (1996), states that:

> The best of Muslims is not he who takes advantage of this life to the extent of losing the future life; neither is the best of the Muslims he who sacrifices the present life in order to gain the future life; the best of the Muslims is he who draws good from both lives. (pp. 97-98)

The vocation of man: adoration of Allah

Making reference to the Koran, the *Shari'a* asserts that the appearance of man on earth was not accidental or lacking purpose. Man's appearance was the execution of a wise divine plan, and achieves the intentions of worshipping and offering testimony to Allah who said:

> I created the jiin and humankind only that they might worship Me. (51:56)

According to the above verse, it is evident "that the worship of Allah is the supreme purpose of the human life" (Al-Naggar 1996, p. 33). Worship is thus the perpetual orientation of Allah by the Muslim, and is central to every thought, behaviour and undertaking.

Providing an explanation of worship, Al-Naggar (1996) comes to the realisation that obedience and humiliation are essential components of worship. Human logic would not see this as a contradiction with the grandeur and sublimity of man because:

> ... in the logic of Allah, there is no greatness and sublimity of man without a total submission and a slavery to Allah. (p. 71)

Furthermore, the Muslim man is to bear witness to the existence of Allah and His prophet Muhammad through faith. Just as the word *Islam* means "the surrender of one's self to Allah," the word *iman*, that is, 'faith' means " As such, the Islamic faith is essentially oriented towards giving witness, for:

> Islam greatly values the concept of giving witness; giving witness to God is the sole worthy attitude that man, a being which is created from mud and blood, can have towards his creator. (Gardet 1967, p. 33; Gardet and Arkoun 1978, p. 18)

Further to managing the earth, the *Shari'a* suggests that man, as a vicar of Allah, must study the signs found in the universe as they in fact are signs from Allah. These signs address the intelligence of man, and as the Koran states:

> Lo! In the creation of the heavens and the earth and (in) the difference of night and day are tokens (of His sovereignty) for men of understanding,

Such as remember Allah, standing, sitting, and reclining [signs], and consider the creation of the heavens and the earth, (and say): Our Lord! Thou createdst not this in vain. Glory be to Thee! Preserve Us from the doom of Fire. (3:190-191)

Nevertheless, one of the first duties of the man who is *gifted with intelligence,* is to learn how to read and ponder on *the signs of Allah* in the universe. Interpreters of the Koranic text have unanimously summoned man to acquire legitimate knowledge, believing that it will confirm within him the word of Allah. Knowledge *(Ilm)* has always been held in the highest regard in Islam (Gardet, 1967). Two *Hadiths* as noted by Gardet (1967), are often quoted to illustrate the expectation of knowledge *(ilm)* in Islam whereby:

> The ink of a religious sciences scholar is more valuable than the blood of the martyr who died, weapons in hand, on the path of God" ...."Seek knowledge, even when it would be in China." (p. 52)

As Allah's vicar, and having received from Him the duty to manage the earth, and being ordered to use his capacity to think and reason, the Muslim man is not called to disdain or ignore the wonders of this world. In fact, he is urged to learn and take advantage of the sciences while bearing in mind that:

> ... Everything will perish save His countenance. His is the command, and unto Him ye will be brought back. (28:88)

Islamic bioethics must then take into account the two truths that concern man: the first being to worship Allah, acknowledging that his existence is bound to Him, as all that he is and all that he has, comes from the Creator; the second truth is that man's reason for being, according to Islamic dogma, is to give witness to the Unique Allah and His messenger, Muhammad. These two truths are thus considered to be the basis of Islamic anthropology, the field in which bioethics should be based and to which it must refer.

In Summary

The concept of man in Islam stems entirely from the Koran. Being composed of both body and spirit, the Muslim is created by God to be superior to the heavens, the earth and the angels. It is from the manner in which he was created that man derives his great value and his dignity. However, in spite of the honour and grandeur bestowed upon him, he is ontologically a frail and perishable creature. Thus, these two realities form the identity of Muslim man.

Additionally, at a conference held in 1974 about "The vision of man in Islam, and the aspiration of man for peace," the Muslim was presented as:

> ... a vicar and responsible; he worships the Merciful; he eats and enjoys the delights and fruits of the earth, according to Allah's *Shari'a* which considers man's buccal (gustatory), sexual and material needs." (*International Council of Churches Symposium* 1974, pp. 109-110)

Furthermore, this vision of man, which is central to every responsibility and right in Islam, is universal, regardless of race, nationality or social rank.

However, Islamic anthropology is based on the relationship between man and Allah. The extent to which it values man and confers upon him dignity, is somewhat questionable. The theoretical inequality between man and woman in Islam challenges the dignity of the human person. Subsequently, Islamic bioethics is based on the teaching of the *Shari'a*, rather than the human person as a creature of Allah.

The Muslim man can only comprehend his existence through Allah, as His vicar, His worshiper, and His faithful servant. His vocation is fulfilled in praising the Lord and being master of the Universe. Ultimately, once the Islamic man confesses that *"God is God, therefore I am"*, a door is opened to consider the human person as the foundation and aim of bioethics (Borrman 1993, p. 40).

Postscript
Convergences and Divergences

Convergences and divergences in the foundations of bioethics

No one can deny the importance of a clear concept of the human person within the realm of bioethics and other areas of practical ethics. Indeed, any right to intervene or interfere with the human body or with human life must be related to this concept. The principle belief that the human being is a creature of God is an intrinsic element of Catholicism and Islam. Furthermore, an interreligious bioethics is only possible with some common understanding of the human person. Nevertheless, the convergences and divergences are a reflection of the anthropological doctrine pertaining to each religion.

Convergences

Both the Catholic Church and Islam consider 'man' to be a creature or creation of God. Starting with this principle, the two religious beliefs concur with regards to the following:

1. Created by God, 'man' is perceived as the masterpiece of creation. This belief provides, for the most part, the reality of 'man' in both religions. 'Man' is a privileged creature of God, depending on Him for existence and life.
2. The Catholic Church and Islam agree that 'man' is distinguished from all other creatures, believing that God Himself breathed His Spirit, into 'man'. As such, the nature of 'man' is sacred and inviolable, as his body is made from the earth, and his spirit which is the principle of life, has been given to him by God.

3. With the unity of body and spirit, 'man' is a fulfilled and living being: a human person brought to life by the principle coming from God. 'Man' therefore is perceived as having dual dimensions which form his purpose and significance: while the union of corporeal and spiritual attributes provides the foundation of human dignity.
4. In both the Catholic and Islamic faiths, each 'man' will be fulfilled through faith and the worship of God. The relationship between God and 'man' is not just the result of 'man's' existence through creation, but it is also a vital relationship founded on his spiritual nature; 'man's' spirit which makes him eternal. From this unique relationship, which is constitutive for man, derives the significance and the value of human life, emphasised as a sacred gift from God. As such, the vocation of the corporeal and spiritual being is fulfilled through the worship and service of God.
5. The Catholic Church and Islam point out the existence of a connection which binds 'man' to the world. It is agreed that the world was created for 'man,' God's favourite creature. Accordingly, 'man' is granted dominion and power over the world and all other creatures.

Divergences

Although the Catholic Church and Islam agree on some aspects regarding the nature and creation of man, there also exist key differences. These include:

1. Both the Bible and Koran describe the creation of 'man' from soil *(turab)* or the earth, however, the creation of Adam is related variously. In the Bible, God created Adam on the sixth day, and was created in His image and

likeness (Gen 1:27). The Koranic account describes the creation of man by *separation* from a pre-existing matter, and through *successive phases* or stages of growth.

2. The Catholic Church points out that *"God created man in the image of himself, in the image of God he created him, male and female he created them"* (Gen 1:27). As such, equality and dignity between man and woman are presupposed: they were created one for the other to cooperate in the work of the Creator, in particular through human procreation.

   The Islamic account does not consider man to be created in Allah's image. Additionally, while woman in Islam is created from man as in the Catholic belief, the Koran states that the position of woman is secondary to man. There is no equality between man and woman, given the ontological view that woman is inferior to man and was created for him. This fundamental difference between the Catholic Church and Islam regarding the concept of woman undermines the question of human rights, the principles of human dignity and equality between all of God's creatures, and promotes sexual discrimination. This significant divergence presents human rights and interreligious bioethics with a major challenge.

3. According to the teaching of the Catholic Church, 'man' exists through Jesus Christ, who teaches the mystery and love of God the Father, revealing Himself to 'man' so that 'man' becomes aware of the magnificence of his vocation. This Christic view presents a singular perspective on Christian anthropology, opening the doors to love and sacrifice. As such, 'man' is deserving of God's vocation, so that he may accordingly fulfil the purpose of human existence.

Conversely, Islamic man was created as a witness of the Unique Allah and His messenger Muhammad, and exists only through a connection with Allah which makes him worthy of being a man. Islamic anthropology proceeds within this relational commitment which must be lived in a quasi-blind obedience to the *Shari'a*.

4. The Catholic Church teaches 'man' to be the master and protector of life, just as God the Creator loves all which He has created. This concept is carried out through a *shared lordship* which is similar to a divine lordship in its commitment to love creation. Accordingly, the sovereignty of 'man' over the universe is not an arbitrary domination, but rather a stewardship which is based on the love, respect and wisdom and recognising the right of all creatures to exist in the manner intended by God.

   Islam teaches a *beneficial lordship* of man over the universe and all living creatures. The *Shari'a* does not determine the conditions of this lordship, but the absence of any form of love between man and Allah's creation is evident. The Islamic viewpoint suggests that the superiority of man over the universe provides sufficient qualification to enable him to manage the earth in a responsible way. Thus, man is able to meet God's expectation of worship, while enjoying the right to benefit from the fruits of the earth to satisfy his buccal, sexual and material needs, in accordance with Allah's *Shari'a*.

'Man' becomes himself when he shows a disposition to accept diversity. However, this acceptance must not compromise either his dignity or the dignity of any human person, male or female. Interreligious bioethics is thus open to religious differences and is derived from them, but it cannot be supported if the fundamental rights of the human being are not promoted and guaranteed by the relevant faith and religion.

Part Two

The Significance of Human Sexuality

Introduction

While being a fundamental component and essential dimension of every human being, sexuality characterises the person, and shapes their sincere engagement in the human condition (Thevenot, 1975). Sexuality determines the person in their "way of being in the world" and imprints the human person as what it is in its activities and relationships with the cosmos, other people and themselves (Durand, 1977; Aubert, 1987). Sexuality, in the context of this discussion, will be examined from a bioethical perspective, rather than through an exhaustive examination of the Catholic and Islamic points of view. Accordingly, in the bioethical context, human sexuality will be addressed through the notions of human corporeality and marriage.

A comparison between the Catholic Church and Islam and their respective teaching regarding human sexuality, is also relevant to an understanding of the anthropological foundations of bioethics. Part One of this book provided the primary step towards this understanding, in its discussion of the concept of 'man.' By comparing the Catholic Church and Islam on sexual ethics, it will establish another facet of the anthropological foundations of bioethics. As such, the question to be raised here is: *is sexuality a subject where the Catholic Church and Islam agree or disagree?*

Therefore, the following chapters will provide an account of each religious perspective: first, chapter 3 discusses the teaching of the Catholic Church, and outlines the Biblical as well as the contemporary teaching of the Magisterium regarding sexuality. Secondly, Chapter 4 examines the Islamic perspective, presenting the Koranic teachings as well as those of some scholars of the *Shari'a*. A presentation of the similarities and differences in thought between the two religions will be the concluding point in our discussion.

Additional resources will be referred to. To capture the Catholic perspective, we will discuss the Apostolic Exhortation of Pope John Paul II, *Familiaris Consortio* (1981), and the Pontifical Council for the Family conference document, *The Truth and Meaning of Human Sexuality* (1995). The Islamic discussion will also make reference to various texts regarding the significance of human sexuality, including *Al-gins fil-qur'an (Sex in the Koran)* (Mahmud, 1994) and *Islam and Moral Sexual Equality* (Aroua, 1990).

3

Bioethics and Sexuality: The Catholic Perspective

According to the Catholic Church, sexuality is a precious gift to human beings from God. This notion is based on the Biblical text, and is expanded by the teachings of the Magisterium.

As we have seen in our discussion thus far, in Christianity and Islam, 'man' has a duality that is both corporeal and spiritual. According to these religions, he is an "I-You" fulfilled as a person through his relationship with others. As an expression of human love, sexuality expresses this need for communion and encounter with another. It is through the body that the human being, man or woman, is manifested and fulfilled as a sexual being. Furthermore, the connection between sexuality and procreation has led to the Catholic bioethical emphasis on both a personalist and responsible vision of human sexuality.

In God's plan for 'man,' sexuality is a way of being which is an essential component of the human person. As such, the reference to sexuality in the Catholic Church:

> ... is not a genital reality but a constitutive dimension of the human being, a power, a potential for love that characterises his entire spiritual and corporeal being and represents a value entrusted to him. (Rocchetta 1993, p. 131)

Sexuality in the Catholic theological tradition

The Church teachings relating to sexuality are based on Sacred Scripture, even though the Scriptures do not include a systemic discourse or formulated set of norms regarding sexuality (Rossi, 1992). The Old Testament provides the first image of human sexuality, presenting it as a fundamental component of being as either man or woman. Referring to the original reality of human sexuality as disclosed in the Old Testament, the New Testament develops its own teaching pertaining to the vocations of matrimony and celibacy.

Sexuality according to the Old Testament

The Old Testament provides both a literal and intrinsic approach to the human being as being both male and female, and as created by God *in his image and to his likeness.* The sexual difference between Adam and Eve is an integral part of their being, for:

> God created man in the image of himself, in the image of God he created him, male and female he created them. (Gen 1:27)

The fact of being in the *image of God* becomes actualised through the polarity of the two sexes, and through the correlativity of their relational existence. Accordingly, man and woman are the embodiment of sexual beings, and exist only as such. Sexuality is not a more or less marginal component, but determines the way of being of the human creature as man or woman, and as *sexual beings* (Piana, 1990; Rossi, 1992).

The human being as either male or female is futile if deprived of a body and sexual specificity, thus sexuality characterises the totality of the human person, and not just the body. In this regard, God's blessing for the first human couple was to:

> ... 'Be fruitful, multiply, fill the earth and subdue it.' (Gen 1:28)

Therefore, the aim of sexuality is human procreation, as well as the realisation of 'man' as a human person. The sexual existence of man and woman finds in marriage a direct and immediate possibility of realisation. God's task to transmit life is thus entrusted to men and women in the form of an engagement to a free and responsible collaboration in God's work (Gilbert, 1974; Rocchetta 1993).

Furthermore, Autiero (1990) explains that the *Song of Songs* in the Old Testament encourages a positive vision of the union of body and soul in the human being, where the manifestation of beauty and human love is expressed through sexual attraction, and lived as a moment of love. Love is thus a requirement of sexuality, and confers a duality on the reproductive dimension: creating unity through the becoming of *"one flesh"* (Gen 2:24), and the creator of human continuity (Gen 1:28). This love is thus derived from a benediction and gift (Vidal, 1996).

Sexuality as a longing for communion

The Yahwist text suggests the original solitude of man, who does not find a companion of the same nature among creatures, or an interlocutor equal to him. For the fulfilment of man, God said:

> It is not right that the man should be alone. I shall make him a helper. (Gen 2:18)

Accordingly, woman was created by God and brought to man to put an end to his solitude. Man's exclamation on seeing the first woman expresses the solitude he had felt and his desire for companionship and life in communion with her. If deprived of this aspect, sexuality will not be authentically fulfilled as it is a promise of encounter and a desire for communion. As such, sexuality is a gift from God which is destined to free the human creature from solitude and to enable it to enter into relationships with others, revealing, at the same time, that sexuality manifests as a man longing for a woman and *vice versa*, as written in the corporeality of human nature (Gilbert, 1977).

In the *General Audience* of 21 November 1979, Pope John Paul II articulates this longing for communion in the text of Genesis 2:23. He asserts that:

> ... femininity finds itself, in a sense, in the presence of masculinity, while masculinity is confirmed through femininity. Precisely the function of sex, which is in a sense, "a constituent part of the person" (not just "an attribute of the person"), proves how deeply man, with all his spiritual solitude, with the never to be repeated uniqueness of his person, is constituted by the body as "he" or "she." The presence of the feminine element, alongside the male element and together with it, signifies an enrichment for man in the whole perspective of his history, including the history of salvation.

Sexuality as a vocation: to give and to receive

The Yahwist text refers to the unity of the flesh, when man and his wife *"become one flesh"* (Gen 2:24). According to Pope John Paul II (*General Audience* of 21 November 1979), this citation defines the bond between the first man and the first woman and provides the perspective of 'man's' earthly future . The sexual act between man and woman is considered as being a full and direct actualisation of *giving and receiving*, and this profoundly characterises their being.

Biblical terminology refers to the sexual act as an act of *knowledge*: it is not only the expression of an encounter of two bodies, but also the communion of two people in which they are able to know who they are. The sexual act is an act of love that is manifested through their mutual sincerity to give and receive and grow in unity. The becoming of *one flesh* is not directly or exclusively orientated towards the act of procreation and the perpetuation of the human species, but rather towards the realisation of a complete communion between man and woman, and illustrates unity by means of the sexual act.

When examining this Biblical position, Rocchetta (1993) claims that sexuality is in fact a call to give, and states:

> Such is the native and fundamental vocation of the human

> creature which is realised through a communion characterised by exchange and giving, receiving and selflessness (altruism). Sexuality is a vocation to realise a modality of existence. The human body expresses this vocation through its structure. Thus the fulfilment of the human person must necessarily go through this mutual motion: from receiving to giving and from giving to receiving. (p. 135)

The creation of the human being attests that the sexual act is one of giving and receiving. The history of creation is marked by the fact that God created man and woman as interlocutors capable of free choice, and thus having the freedom to answer His commandments with a "yes" or "no." As such, sexuality is entrusted to the freedom of human beings and should accordingly be handled responsibly.

Putting aside any liberal or positive points of view about sexuality, love and human procreation, the Old Testament puts before us the weaknesses and limits of human sexuality. The human person is exposed to sexual temptation, infidelity and other sins that alter the purpose of the sexual act, and cause childbirth to be painful (Autiero, 1990). The Old Testament also presents the reality of sexual differentiation into male and female as intended by God, who confirmed His positive judgement regarding the order of creation:" God saw all he had made, and indeed it was very good" (Gen 1:31).

Sexuality according to the New Testament

The New Testament does not present Jesus as teaching extensively on sexuality . He mainly refers to the image of man and woman as described in the Old Testament (Mk 10:6 and Mt 19:4). Evidently, sexuality is not elaborated in the New Testament which maintains that it is a gift from God to 'man': it is neither an evil, nor a malediction, nor a function of the human being, but it is his way (his manner) of being (Autiero, 1990).

In the Gospels of Mark (10:6-9) and Matthew (19:4-6), Jesus

teaches that the creative love of God establishes the basis of love which exists between man and woman. Sexuality is the sign and instrument whereby the creative love of God is perceptible in human love. Yet when Jesus speaks of adultery, he not only condemns the act, but also denounces it as contrary to the true fulfilment of sexuality (Mt 5:27-28). Moreover, the sincerity of a heart becomes the essential prerequisite of an authentic intent to engage in the sexual act, thus becoming an expression of love and communion. This reality of love and communion is a call to live in a transparency where man and woman can recognise themselves through the body of the other, while respecting it with dignity. The gaze then, is one of respect and not sexual domination. Sexuality then, is relevant to the vocation of human being, and it is only through true transparency that it fulfills its purpose (Rossi, 1992).

St Paul provides a slightly different vision of sexuality. In his first letter to the Corinthians (1 Cor 7:8-9), St Paul emphasises celibacy and provides a negative impression of sexuality. In that same letter, St Paul prompts the Corinthians to regard the human body as having its own dignity and thus to be respected (1 Cor 5:12-20). This teaches those who would confuse freedom with libertinism that the human body is not an object or instrument. It is in fact an expression of the person, and ultimately the temple of the divine Presence, where the humanity of 'man' is reinforced (John Paul II, 1985; MacDonald, 1991).

Sexuality, in both the Old and New Testaments, maintains an affirmation of two key concepts:

- From creation, sexuality is seen as being a gift which the hands of God have placed in the hands of human beings, to be assumed and used for its intrinsic purpose. This perspective indicates that sexuality is to be used in its integrity, and not made into a taboo or a myth.

- Sexuality in the Bible can only be comprehended in the context of a covenant. Conjugal love is in fact viewed as a sign of the love that Yahweh had for Israel. Sexuality, then, is a constitutive dimension of human love which symbolises a larger reality , that is, the revelation of God's love through Jesus Christ who made human love partake in the mystery of God. Therefore, "the human *eros* is inserted in the *agape* which is in itself the nature of God" (Penna 1984, p. 40).

Similarly and as per the Sacred Scriptures, sexuality may become an extraordinary source of growth and altruism, as long as it is orientated towards giving and receiving *the gift* and *the agape* (selfless love), which are received according to the Creator and Saviour's will. Sexuality may also become a destructive and narcissistic act if used for power, pleasure and egocentricity, ignoring God's will.

Häring (1989) provides a concluding thought regarding sexuality in the Sacred Scriptures, stating:

> Sexuality has been thought of in this manner by the only God and Creator. The creative and redemptive love of God has just been bestowed upon all men of all epochs; we are aware that not only men and women, in their reciprocity and bipolarity, have been created to the image and likeness of God; but we are also aware that the perfect image of the invisible God is Jesus Christ. Thus we can only conceive sexuality through the perspective of redeemed love. Through this love we reach an integrated vision of sexuality, highlighted by the fact that God is love. And therefore the sexual dimension of man and woman finds redemption and fulfilment in the light of this truth. (pp. 613-614)

Sexuality in the contemporary Magisterium

It is evident that the Biblical account of sexuality finds the original reality of sexuality engrained within the human person, male and female. It is their natural vocation to love and communicate in the acknowledgement of God, the source of human life, that establishes the norm of ethical behaviour. The following account is not an in depth examination of sexuality as discussed in the Magisterium, but only a brief account of the recent teaching of the Church.

Sexuality and marriage

The teaching of the Catholic Church does not offer a complete discourse about sexuality. However, the subject of marriage as it relates to sexuality is the exception, as it is an essential correlation for anthropological observations and thus Catholic bioethics. To position sexuality as an exclusive expression of human love within a marriage, the declaration of the Pontifical Council for The Family, *The Truth and Meaning of Human Sexuality* (1995), confirms that:

> When such love exists in marriage, self-giving expresses, through the body, the complementarity and totality of the gift. Married love thus becomes a power which enriches persons and makes them grow and, at the same time, it contributes to building up the civilization of love. But when the sense and meaning of gift is lacking in sexuality, a "civilization of things and not of persons" takes over, "a civilization in which persons are used in the same way as things are used." (Vatican City, 8 December 1995)

In order to confirm the reality of sexuality as a reciprocal gift of man and woman within marriage, the Apostolic Exhortation *Familiaris Consortio*, of Pope John Paul II (1981) states:

> The only "place" in which this self-giving in its whole truth is made possible is marriage, the covenant of conjugal love

> freely and consciously chosen, whereby man and woman accept the intimate community of life and love willed by God Himself which only in this light manifests its true meaning. (11)

However:

> While it is normal and good for physical union to be the natural consequence of a true and exclusive love, it is certain that sexuality, within marriage as well as celibacy, can be raised beyond its biological purposes and consciously directed towards authentic human values: freedom, beauty, tenderness, brotherly love. (Synode Diocésain de Suisse Romande 1975, p. 218)

While recalling the origins of human existence in the Sacred Scriptures as a sexual existence, sexuality in the Magisterium can be presented through three notions: a *constitutive dimension* of the person, a *total self-giving*, and as a *nostalgic desire of the other*. Moreover, the ability to procreate that God has entrusted to man and woman through a special benediction, has great significance in the Church (Franck, 1980).

The Sacred Congregation for Catholic Education in their *Educational Guidance In Human Love* (1984) stresses the connection between sexuality and procreation:

> Sexual intercourse, ordained towards procreation, is the maximum expression on the physical level of the communion of love of the married. Divorced from this context of reciprocal gift – a reality which the Christian enjoys, sustained and enriched in a particular way by the grace of God it loses its significance, exposes the selfishness of the individual, and is a moral disorder. (5)

The Catholic understanding of sexuality and procreation through conjugal union determines the position of the Church on medically assisted procreation, and will be examined in the forthcoming Volume II.

Sexuality as a constitutive dimension of the human person

In Catholicism, the harmonious development of the human personality involves the spiritual-corporeal dimensions of 'man.' For instance the Sacred Congregation for Catholic Education states:

> Sexuality is a fundamental component of personality, one of its modes of being, of manifestation, of communicating with others, of feeling, of expressing and of living human love. Therefore it is an integral part of the development of the personality ... (Sacred Congregation for Catholic Education 1984, 4)

Likewise, the *Catechism of the Catholic Church* (1995) associates sexuality with the unity of the human being. Accordingly, the objective of the sexual act is to procreate and to express marital love because:

> Sexuality affects all aspects of the human person in the unity of his body and soul. It especially concerns affectivity, the capacity to love and to procreate, and in a more general way the aptitude for forming bonds of communion with others. (2332)

Sexuality then, reflects this bond of communion between man and woman within the framework of marriage. The *Catechism of the Catholic Church* defines marriage as a sacrament of union with Christ, and as an alliance between man and woman. Thus,

> Sexuality is ordered to the conjugal love of man and woman. In marriage the physical intimacy of the spouses becomes a sign and pledge of spiritual communion. Marriage bonds between baptized persons are sanctified by the sacrament. (2360)

Furthermore, the Sacred Congregation for the Doctrine of Faith explains in *Persona Humana* (1975) how the sexual act characterises the human person, stating that:

> In fact it is from sex that the human person receives the characteristics which, on the biological, psychological and spiritual levels, make that person a man or a woman, and thereby largely condition his or her progress towards maturity and insertion into society. (1)

According to the above statement, sexuality is to be regarded as a constitutive manner of being that is inscribed in the totality of the human person, and determines the difference between man and woman on several levels, from their physical configuration, to their state of mind and spiritual life. Thus, Pope John Paul II states in *Familiaris Consortio* (1981) that:

> ... sexuality, by means of which man and woman give themselves to one another through the acts which are proper and exclusive to spouses, is by no means something purely biological, but concerns the innermost being of the human person as such. (11)

The human person as a whole is engaged through their sexuality, and is orientated towards the reciprocal existence of mutually *giving and receiving* with others. Accordingly, those who reject the physical act of sex do not necessarily reject sexuality. They do not reject their being as man and woman who are called to communion, or to take part in *giving and receiving* throughout their lives.

Sexuality as a total self-giving

Sexuality does not merely characterise the human being as a sexual being, it is also an innate and fundamental human expression of their vocation to communion and love. It fulfils its purpose when it leads both man and woman through a life of love and communion, to the vocation of consecrated life or to that of marriage. According to the Pontifical Council for The Family:

> When love is lived out in marriage, it includes and surpasses

friendship. Love between a man and woman is achieved when they give themselves totally, each in turn according to their own masculinity and femininity ... (1995, 14)

Conjugal love is expressed through the reciprocal attraction of two wills and the disposition of total self-giving of two people (*Gaudium et Spes*, 49). Conversely, chastity is also a means to a self-giving life. Thus the Pontifical Council for The Family (1995) affirms that:

> Chastity is the joyous affirmation of someone who knows how to live self-giving, free from any form of self-centred slavery...The chaste person is not self-centred, not involved in selfish relationships with other people. Chastity makes the personality harmonious. It matures it and fills it with inner peace. (14)

Celibacy for the sake of the Kingdom of Heaven is thus neither an individual exercising self-control over instinct, nor a Manichaeism is hostile to sexuality, nor revulsion against marriage, but rather the particular expression of an unconditional gift to Christ. Accordingly, if a man or woman – married or consecrated – is not able to show love and communion, they are not capable of living the profound meaning of their sexuality. Hoeffner (1973) expands on this subject, saying that whoever attempts an explanation of sexuality in the context of faith must not neglect to mention celibacy for the sake of the Kingdom of Heaven. Marriage and celibacy are bound closely together. They draw their existence from the mystery of the Church, and denote the things to come. A sexuality that is lived in full should bear the fruits of availability to others, altruism, self-sacrifice, kindheartedness, serenity and the responsible fulfilment of one's duties. In other words:

> Sexuality, oriented, elevated and integrated by love acquires truly human quality. Prepared by biological and psychological development, it grows harmoniously and is achieved in the

full sense only with the realisation of affective maturity, which manifests itself in unselfish love and in the total gift of self. (Sacred Congregation for Catholic Education 1984, 6)

Sgreccia (1994) has elaborated on this theme, stating that sexuality is not the equivalent of exercising genitality. As such, a differentiation must be made between relations between sexes and genital sexual relations . 'Relations between sexes' refers to every relation between individuals from the opposite sex, whether it is friendship, regard or affection, without resulting in genital sexual relations. On the other hand, genital sexual relations take place between a man and a woman where there is mutual and complete personal gift through genital sexual union. It is essential to distinguish between the two, given that exercising genitality is not the unique means of expression as man or woman. Moreover, being a man does not necessarily entail being a husband or father, neither does being a woman crucially mean wife or mother.

In God's original plan, sexuality is, in essence, the power of love and the promise of communion. Sexuality in itself is then destined to pave the way for the human person to exit the strict circle of the individual "I," and be open to encounters with others, with "you," based on the capacity of communion and love. *Familiaris Consortio*, of Pope John Paul II (1981), states that such a communion is:

> ... the natural complementarity that exists between man and woman, and is nurtured through the personal willingness of the spouses to share their entire life-project, what they have and what they are: for this reason such communion is the fruit and the sign of a profoundly human need. (19)

The Magisterium emphasises that "human sexuality is thus a good" (The Pontifical Council for The Family 1995, 11) and a value entrusted to responsibility of humanity. However, it is not an outlet freely available to satisfy physical needs, but rather a *value* related to the gift of life. In the consecrated life, sexuality also expresses the giving of self to Jesus Christ who is full of love for humanity. Through Jesus, communion is discovered and actualised in the reciprocal gift of the human life, for "human life is a gift received in order then to be given as a gift" (Pope John Paul II 1995, 92). The Catholic Church then views sexuality as an engagement to overcome the self-centredness hidden within the human heart, and to develop altruism and generosity.

Sexuality as a nostalgic desire for the Other
According to the Catholic Church, sexuality exceeds the biological reality that differentiates between male and female: it is takes the individual beyond their personal psychology, character and physical makeup, because it carries an inexhaustible and ceaseless call to transcendence. This call is based on two fundamental factors, being the limits of sexuality and the disposition towards infinity inscribed in the heart of each human being "called to become a partaker of God's life" (Pope John Paul II *General Audience* of 21 November 1979). The exercise of sexuality then defines the innate limit of every human reality and every inter-personal relation; if it is life (*bios*, observing that *bios* is inextricably linked with love or *eros*) it is also death (*thanatos*); if it is wealth, it is also poverty.

Sexuality is inevitably linked to our existence in this world. The human heart preserves the need for transcendence and the desire or "nostalgia" for an infinite love and a complete and unlimited communion. The human creature, as an image of the infinite God, longs for a realisation that surpasses its solely historical actualisation and thus seeks a realisation in God. Therefore, sexuality is subject to the same law as the human condition, and is both a reminder and a desire for full union with the God of life and love (Rocchetta, 1993).

Being created in God's image, 'man' is therefore created to love. This reality was revealed in the First Letter of John (4:8) in the New

Testament at the same time as the mystery of the intra-Trinitarian life: "... *God is love"* and he lives in himself a mystery of personal communion and love. By creating man and woman in his image, and providentially supplying the human vocation to form a single pair and to procreate, God bestows upon us both the capacity and the responsibility to desire and achieve communion and love. The *Catechism of the Catholic Church* (1995) states that this vocation is expressed, but not exclusively, through:

> Sexuality, by means of which man and woman give themselves to one another through the acts which are proper and exclusive to spouses ... (2361)

Furthermore, without love, the human being is not able to fulfil their "fundamental and innate vocation." (*Catechism of the Catholic Church* 1995, 2392)

According to Pope John Paul II in *Familiaris Consortio* (1981, 9 and 11), the theological foundation of 'man' and his particular vocation relates to the eternal mystery of the person that has been created in the image of God, and is incarnated in the visible and corporeal manifestation of the human person through masculinity and femininity.

This facet of sexuality, a call to altruistic love and communion, can only be understood through the love revealed by Jesus Christ. This love reveals to 'man' his true identity, as:

> ... "Christ the new Adam, in the very revelation of the mystery of the Father and of his love, fully reveals man to himself and brings to light his most high calling." (Pontifical Council for The Family 1995, 9)

Regardless of the demands of such love, it establishes the true good of 'man.' As such, Pope John Paul II in his *General Audience* of 16 January 1980, states that love is true when it creates the good within people and communities, and then offers that good to all other people.

The separation of sexuality and love is the most serious flaw in today's culture and contradicts the Catholic concept of sexuality. When it is performed within the context of an authentic communion of love the sexual act is the complete realisation of the person. To overcome and prevent the schism of sexuality and true love, the Sacred Congregation for Catholic Education places an emphasis on sex education (22 October 1983, Article 5), as both a right and a duty for parents and educational centres. In *Familiaris Consortio* (1981), Pope John Paul II explains the connection between the necessity of sex education and personal morality, saying:

> In view of the close links between the sexual dimension of the person and his or her ethical values, education must bring the children to a knowledge of and respect for the moral norms as the necessary and highly valuable guarantee for responsible personal growth in human sexuality. (37)

The irresponsible depersonalisation of sexual practices is regarded as inhumane, hence the requirement for responsible sex education. Accordingly, responsibility for sexual engagement seems to be necessary to enable each person to be aware and be capable of self-determination, so that sexual energy and desires are channelled according to that person's vocation and free choice.

In Summary

Sexuality, according to Catholicism, is "a dimension of the human person and a confirmation of the being" (Piana 1994, p.897). It is in effect 'good' like all that was created and intended by God, who confers life and meaning, and maintains the existence of all living creatures. Human sexuality is not entrusted to each person to engage in as they please, but rather to recognise and discover the true meaning of God's divine will. To be totally and truly human, sexuality must therefore take place in conjugal life, emphasising the value of love and being loved.

The purpose of the sexual act is only realised when it is used to express the reciprocal feeling of love, no matter the obstacles to that love. It is, paradoxically, an expression where differences are experienced in the most intimate manner. Sexuality is orientated as a form of interpersonal dialogue and thus contributes to the integral maturity of the human being, allowing each person to offer their self as a gift of love. It is related to the fertilisation and transmission of life, and is therefore an act that must remain faithful to that purpose.

The Magisterium of the Catholic Church, notes that the human person is capable of expressing different forms of love, such as *superior love* that is not the lustful desire that only seeks to satisfy sexual appetites, but is also a love that encompasses friendship, the offering of oneself as an oblation (self-offering), self-giving, and grants the person the ability to know love. Similarly, the Magisterium discusses chastity as an undertaking which *walks in the footsteps of Christ*, realising the integration of sexuality in the human person in a manner that includes acquiring the discipline of self-control.

Hence, every baptised person is called to lead a chaste life, as part of their own daily way of life. Chastity thus becomes a virtue to be lived partially in conjugal life and fully in consecrated life (*Catechism of the Catholic Church* 1995, 2394-2395). Furthermore, sexuality is seen as an expression of a generous love that is in the likeness of God's love, for love is the only virtue that leads to communion between people, and which considers the 'good' of others as their own. The relation between love and human sexuality is clarified when we take into consideration that 'man' is called to love and that human sexuality is a 'good' (Pontifical Council for The Family 1995, 10 and 11).

4

Bioethics and Sexuality: The Islamic Perspective

In Islam, sexuality is a large constitutive component of human and social life, to the point where the Koran and the *Shari'a* describe sexual activity in its most intimate detail (Aroua, 1990). Islam perceives sexuality as a universal necessity of life. Bousquet (1990) confirms this, stating:

> Islam is frankly and openly propitious to the pleasures of the flesh as such, without any incidental consideration. However, this propitiousness is not without its restrictions. Islam marks boundaries in this domain considering that the Muslim is not to commit the crime-sin of *zina* (adultery). (p. 49)

Accordingly, Islamic bioethics tends to direct the practice of sexuality according to the well defined paths of the *Shari'a*, where "marriage as a legitimate form of communal life must grant a fair place to the practice of sexual relations" (Balic 1991, p. 551). Bioethics and sexuality in Islam are strongly related to the Islamic theological tradition and to the contents of the contemporary *Shari'a*.

Sexuality in the Islamic theological tradition

Sexuality has a privileged status in Islam. The Koranic verses speak of sexuality, and assert the right to enjoy sexual pleasures. Sexual ethics is based on the example as set by the Prophet of Islam, whose irreproachability was raised to the status of dogma. Every Muslim is urged to follow his example. The Koran also provides the principle basis of the *Shari'a* teachings regarding sexuality.

Sexuality according to the Koran

The term *gins*, meaning sex or sexuality, cannot be found in the Koran (Ibrahim, 1994). Regardless, sexuality and the sexual relationship between a man and a woman has an important place in the Koran, as it does in Islam. A *Hadith* asserts without hesitation that marriage, where sexuality is experienced, represents "half of the religion" (Al-Saar, 1990; Bouhdiba, 1996). When referring to sexuality, the Koran uses the term *nikah*, translated by the term coitus, which becomes legal through the contract of marriage *(keetab)*. The term *nikah* can be found 23 times in the Koran (e.g. 4:3, 4:22, 24:3, 24:32-33, 2:221), to encourage Muslims to marry and procreate (Ibrahim, 1994).

Sexuality inscribed into human nature

Muslims maintain that the Koran prescribes all the basic principles that define and outline the circumstances and manner of sexual relations between man and woman (Aroura, 1990).

Three core principles are pointed to, the first of which highlights the existence of sexually complementary couples, that is, male and female couples. The Koran stipulates this principle as a universal law (Bouhdiba, 1986) in verse 51:49 where it is stated that "And all things We have created by pairs." Aroua (1990) explains this as an Islamic principle where:

> ... sexuality is inscribed in the nature of things that is in the order wanted by Allah. This is why it is integrated in morals at the same time as a necessity, right and duty. It is recognised and accepted in all its dimensions: biological when it is related to reproduction, psychological when it leads to desire and affection and moral each time it implicates reciprocal and common duties. (p. 69)

Rahman (1987) agrees that the Koran provides a universal law, stating that:

> Here and elsewhere, this verse leaves a strong impression that sex represents a universal law. Sex in humans, therefore, is only a special case of this universal phenomenon. (p. 118)

The second principle relating to sexuality is the physiological differences between the first couple, which thus highlights the resulting biological purpose of reproduction and multiplication of the human species (Aroua, 1990). The applicable Koranic verses state:

> O mankind! Be careful of your duty to your Lord Who created you from a single soul and from it created its mate and from them twain hath spread abroad a multitude of men and women. (4:1)
>
> He it is who did create you from a single soul, and therefrom did make his mate that he might take rest in her. (7:189)

Accordingly, human creation originated with two beings of common origin to fulfil the purpose of increasing humankind. Yet they were distinct and complementary, one of the masculine sex and one of the feminine sex. In this light, the Koranic and Biblical verse are alike: "male and female He created them."

The third and final principle refers to the relationship between a man and a woman, clarifying the role of each. The Koran states:

> And of His signs is this: He created for you helpmeets from yourselves that ye might find rest in them, and He ordained between you love and mercy. Lo, herein indeed are portents for folk who reflect . (30:21)

Accordingly, man and woman are made for each other, and thus give themselves to one another.

Sexuality in the man-woman relationship

The Koran clarifies the relationship between man and woman in particular verse 2:223, stating that:

> Your women are a tilth for you (to cultivate) so go to your tilth as ye will, and send (good deeds) before you for your souls, and fear Allah, and know that ye will (one day) meet Him.

According to the above, the relationship between a man and a woman relies on man and his will. Thus, the female is subordinate, particularly in a sexual relationship. This subordinate position of the woman is clear in the above Koranic verse, which forms the basis of the position in the *Shari'a*. (Bouhdiba 1986).

Sexuality in the contemporary *Shari'a*

Whilst being based upon the Koran, the *Shari'a* emphasises the purpose for which sexual *power* is created as an instinct intrinsic to the man. The question to bear in mind is whether or not sexual instinct in the Islamic context is primarily aimed towards physical pleasure, while procreation is of secondary importance. Islam's answer to this is aligned to the viewpoint of Catholicism, which prohibits and condemns all aspects of fornication and adultery. The Koran condemns fornication as an offense against Allah's will, and deems it punishable by a hundred whiplashes (24:2-3). As for adultery, the *Shari'a* stipulates further punishment when the culprits are married: adultery is punishable by death, by stoning, for the man and the woman (as it was in the Old Testament) (Bouhdiba, 1986; Borrmans, 1994). The *Shari'a* also encourages marriage and specifies the modalities of matrimonial sexuality.

Sexuality and marriage

In Islam, the sexual act is prohibited outside of marriage or legal concubinage. The *Shari'a* speaks of sexuality within and outside of marriage, without emphasising concubinage thus:

> In its Shari'a, Islam has clearly defined the modes of sexuality

within marriage so that it would be respected, while precising what is permitted and forbidden. (Al-Saar 1990, p. 48)

Furthermore:

Every sexual relation must then be preceded by a public celebration of the marriage contract. (Aroua 1990, pp. 76-77)

Fazlur (1987) discusses this particular point, and offers a definition of marriage as an appropriate human institution, in which:

... human sex life exhibits characteristics that are unique in the animal kingdom: the institution of marriage and the family. Pre-Islamic Arabia had an institution of "free love" (*khidn*, plural *akhdan*, "partners in free love") which the Koran terminated (4:25 and 5:5) in favour of marital arrangement. (p. 118)

Yet to claim that Islamic law exclusively allows sexual relations within marriage, is not entirely accurate. Islam also allows the practice of sexuality when in the situation of legal concubinage:

There are two licit ways to satisfy the sexual instinct, marriage and legal concubinage between a man and his female servant (70:6). For a married Muslim, there is no "moral" inconvenience for him to take, in addition to his wife [or wives], one or several concubines, following the example of the Prophet Muhammad. (Bousquet 1990, p. 109-110)

The Islamic tradition speaks of the Prophet Muhammad, the impeccable man (Bousquet, 1990) who levied beautiful girls from out of booty received, and distributed them to the father of one of his wives, and to the husbands of two of his daughters. Islam allows polygamy, that is, any Muslim man (provided he is eligible for marriage) is allowed to have up to four wives at any given time. This is still tolerated and legally recognised in the majority of Islamic countries, except for Turkey and Tunisia at the time of writing (Borrmans, 1994).

Nonetheless, the primary purpose of marriage in Islam is the practice of sexuality and the satisfaction of physical instincts. Procreation is not of primary concern, as it is in the tradition of the Church. It is within this context that the first article of the *Moroccan Code of Personal Status* (1957-1958) is to be understood, where it states:

> Marriage is a legal contract of durable and reciprocal union and attachment between a man and a woman. Under the guidance of the husband, the exercise of sexuality and chastity should occur, as well as the multiplication of the nation's numbers, through the creation of families. (Borrmans 1994, p. 3)

Within Islam, the purpose of marriage has been somewhat changed recently, for in the *Universal Islamic Declaration of Human Rights* (19 September 1981), article 19a states that:

> Marriage in the Islamic context is a recognised right of every human being. It is the legitimate way, as per Islamic law, to establish a family and ensure descendants, and keeping personal chastity. Every one of the spouses has equivalent rights and duties as particularly stipulated by Islamic law.

Accordingly, marriage in Islam is an established right for every Muslim. Divine law established it as the legitimate means to establish a family (Abu-Sahlieh, 1994).

Sexuality, the person and coitus (nikah)

As previously stated, the Koran refers to the sexual act as coitus *(nikah)*. According to the Koran, Allah legislated for this act:

> And all married women (are forbidden unto you save those captives) whom your right hands possess. It is a decree of Allah for you. Lawful unto you are all beyond those mentioned, so that ye seek them with your wealth in honest wedlock, not debauchery. And those of whom ye seek

content (by marrying them), give unto them their portions as a duty. And there is no sin for you in what ye do by mutual agreement after the duty (hath been done). Lo! Allah is ever Knowing and Wise. (4:24)

It is obvious then, that the sexual act is illicit without a marriage contract.

Accordingly, the act of coitus *(nikah)* becomes both a law and a duty, provided that the Muslim man has the sexual desire and is ready for marriage. Coitus *(nikah)* is not only a part of the Muslim man's life on earth, but it is at the core of the Muslim man's life in the Islamic paradise. Many verses of the Koran according to Bousquet (1990), depict the sexual relations of the Muslim faithful with the *houris* in paradise. However, the man is required to be capable of self-control and not commit adultery, which is strictly forbidden by Islam as stated in the Koran (25:68-70). Even though celibacy is not encouraged in Islam, the sexual act cannot be enacted with just any woman. Man is not permitted to marry a woman who does not believe in either of the celestial or monotheistic religions, or who is betrothed to another man (Al-Saar, 1990).

According to the *Shari'a*, a couple is not permitted to perform the sexual act in any manner that they may please. They must respect and follow certain laws and norms (Bouhdiba, 1986). For example, prior to the first sexual encounter between husband and wife, they are both required to kneel twice while reading verses from the Koran. Another requirement in the Koran (7:189) is that the man must cover the body of the woman with his own body, as she lies beneath him. In fact, this position during the course of the sexual act is the only one permitted by Islam. However, there is some ambiguity regarding sexual positioning, as another Koranic verse allows the performance of the sexual act according to the will and pleasure of the man, stating "women are a tilth for you (to cultivate) so go to your tilth as ye will" (2:223). In this verse, man is free to exercise sexuality when, where and how he pleases, but in adherence to the instructions of the *Shari'a*. Sodomy between a man and his wife is prohibited, and so too is intercourse during a woman's period, Ramadan, pilgrimage to Mecca, and spiritual retreat in mosques (Al-Saar, 1990). However, the Koran encourages the man to sexually satisfy his wife. Also, a man who divorces his wife by pronouncing the divorce formula three times is unable to remarry her afterwards unless she weds another man and consummates that marriage (Al-Saar, 1990). This is a fact corroborated in the Koran: "if he hath divorced her (the third time), then she is not lawful unto him thereafter until she hath wedded another husband" (2:230).

The Islamic anthropological perspective on sexuality seems to be practically non-existent. As sexual beings, the man and woman experience an encounter or a state of physical pleasure, and not necessarily an act to express their love. This being so, the sexual act is reduced to being an outlet to satisfy sexual instincts, predominantly those of the male. This raises the question of whether sexuality is an equal component and right of the human person as male and female.

Coitus (nikah): satisfying man's desire

In the Islamic context, coitus *(nikah)* is the masculine sexual act, providing the male with possession of the female body. This is reiterated by Ibrahim (1994) who sates that,

> During the *nikah*, there is an elevation of the man above the woman who must be under him, for the authority of man over woman in general is also cemented at this level where he dominates her with his body. In this way, man lives sex with a woman not only enjoying her body, but also with his presence; this means that he has a complete and active presence, whereas the presence of the woman is merely corporeal while she is absent in her being and humanity." (pp. 62-63)

According to the *Shari'a*, sexuality is limited to a relationship between one male and a defined number of women (Ibrahim, 1994). The woman remains the source of enjoyment and pleasure for the male, with her body being a place of sexual relief for him and the object of his carnal passion. Man is therefore free to enjoy the female body, as opposed to a woman who is an independent being. As Bouhdiba, (1986) says: "The authority of the man over the woman goes as far as to negate her being, which leads to the perception of the woman being the property of the man" (p.24).

The Koran provides the foundations of these teachings, stating:

> Men are in charge of women, because Allah hath made the one of them to excel the other, and because they spend of their property (for the support of women). So good women are the obedient, guarding in secret that which Allah hath guarded. As for those from whom ye fear rebellion, admonish them and banish them to beds apart, and scourge them. Then if they obey you, seek not a way against them. (4:34)

The above verse refers to the explicit superiority of the man over woman, whilst considering the woman as the private property and a source of pleasure for the man. Thus the text would indicate that the woman in Islam may live stripped of dignity and autonomy.

Sexuality in Islam is evidently reduced to an act of physical, sensual and genital pleasure. It is a man's pleasure that is related to the sexual act with a woman for purposes of procreation. Once fertilisation has been achieved, the male's role is displaced. Women then generally assume the responsibility of childbirth, and educating the child. Ibrahim (1994) summarises the view of sexuality in Islam by stating:

> It seems that sexual activity in Islam according to the Koran is masculine, for man is the origin and chief. He leads this sexual activity with an authoritarian presence to which woman must be subdued (2:228). In spite of the existence

of proofs that certify the common origins of man and woman (4:1), the privileges given to man have confirmed the negative image of the woman; imperfection, inaptitude and incompetence. In a word, they have proved that she is but an object of sexual pleasure for man, or a corporeal favour for him. Thus man knows love only through sexual relation where the feminine body is being sexually dominated. Even where love exists, sexual desire remains overriding. (p. 151)

It is important to make mention of the sexual pleasure in the Muslim paradise where the faithful are destined, and where a man will have the strength of a hundred men in feeding, drinking and especially sexual pleasure. In fact, a man may be able to have intercourse with seventy virgins a day with unrelenting desire and passion. Thus, even paradise is dominated by the male's sexual activity.

Aroua (1990) however, rejects the idea of female inferiority in Islam, arguing that the bonds between man and woman are first and foremost governed by a fundamental principle of reciprocity. In fact, the Koran states that:

And they (women) have rights similar to those (of men) over them in kindness, and men are a degree above them. (2:228)

The *degree of advantage* mentioned, is further explained when the Koran clarifies the role of man as being:

... in charge of women, because Allah hath made the one of them to excel the other, and because they spend of their property (for the support of women). (4:34)

Accordingly, the intent of the above stated verses is to emphasise the necessity of order and harmony in a relationship that is based on respect and devotion between a man and woman (Aroua, 1990).

Furthermore, Bouhdiba (1986) states that "the woman is a biological capital, and leaving it to be unproductive is impermissible"

(p. 112). This statement highlightsan Islamic view of women reducing her being to the task of reproductivity.

It is also worthwhile noting the "marriages for pleasure", i.e. *al-mutaa* and *al-urfa*. *Al-mutaa* marriages are common amongst Shiite Muslims, and *al-urfa* marriages are common amongst Sunni Muslims. These types of marriages are for a pre-determined amount of money and period of time, for example an hour, after which the marriage is automatically annulled (Al-Saar, 1990).

Sexuality: a necessity and duty of man

The necessity of having an active sexual life and satisfying sexual instincts justifies the purpose for which Allah has granted man his sexual power. This reality is highlighted by Assaf (1991) who states:

> Allah has created man on earth to be His vicar in the construction of the earth. This task may only be realised through the continuity of life and conservation of the human species on earth. For this reason, Allah has created an array of instincts in man, including sexual instinct among others, to ensure the preservation of the species. Sexual instinct in man is a potent power that requires to play its role and to be satisfied ... man would not be capable of fulfilling the mission for which Allah has created him if he did not have instincts, orientating him towards pleasures and desires in order to take what is good and necessary to him. (pp. 74-76)

From the above, we understand that the Muslim *Shari'a* in general, does not accept sexual mortification: Allah in his divine wisdom created man with sexual drives and instincts. It is thus inconceivable that after having been created in such a way, man be asked to ignore sexual drives or to mortify them, as procreation and life inevitably stem from man's sexual instinct. However, some Islamic scholars have a view about sexuality, e.g. Ibn Qayyiem (1974) affirms that sexuality is not a necessary need as are eating or drinking. Therefore, man can live his life without woman and marriage. A balanced Islamic view is also noted where Assaf (1991) states in this regard that

> ... the stance of the Shari'a towards sexual instincts is well balanced, that is, it does not accept abuse and is against humiliation or mortification. In a word, it insists upon a balanced adjustment. (p. 74)

Islamic sexual morals also address chastity *(ihsan)* which is considered to be one of the norms in the relationship that exists between the sexes. The *Shari'a* advocates chastity and decency outside of lawful marriage (Fazlur, 1987), condemning what are considered to be ostentatious or enhanced displays such as sauntering, wearing loud clothing or applying cosmetics with the aim of attracting sexual interest and provoking desires (Aroua, 1990).

Al-Qaradhawi (1994) supports the opinion of Assaf (1991) regarding the creation of the earth and the mission of man as a being created with sexual instinct to procreate and preserve life. However, Al-Qaradhawi (1994) points out that man with his sexual instinct, must adopt one of the three following attitudes:

- Eliminate moral or religious limits to sexual instincts, and so display an animalistic decadence, which is opposed to Islamic thought.
- Repress sexual instincts through a monastic and ascetic life. This is contradictory to Allah's wisdom creating in man the sexual instinct to procreate and conserve life.
- Maintain a balanced stance that sets the boundaries to sexual instincts, which is the position of Islam, creating through the *Shari'a* a moral frame where there is neither repression nor libertinism.

Furthermore, Al-Qaradhawi (1994) states that Islam is against any form of consecrated life and celibacy, prohibiting sexual practices outside of marriage and legal concubinage. The *Shari'a* does however emphasise the value of chastity and abstinence between spouses during the month of Ramadan, and when taking part in the pilgrimage to Mecca.

It follows then, that the creation of sexual instinct in man, according to the *Shari'a*, is dependent on Allah allowing his vicar *(khalifa)* to enjoy the satisfaction of his sexual desires. The mission entrusted to the vicar can only be accomplished when humankind maintains its life and grows on earth, procreating, in accordance with Islamic law.

In Summary

Islam requires that the sexual act take place within marriage or legal concubinage, where the rights of both spouses are assured. In the understanding and teaching of Islam, prostitution, pre-marital or extra-marital relations, and any type of liberal union are prohibited. Furthermore, Islam provides a detailed and explicit description of the proper practice in any sexual relationship, so that man can achieve sexual satisfaction.

As such, all Muslims regard "sexuality as a natural phenomenon [that] is inseparable from the life created by Allah. Therefore it must not be ignored, degraded or condemned" (Aroua 1990, p. 264), but engaged in as a means to pleasure and procreation. Sexual pleasure is attained during the act of coitus *(nikah)*, and during man's domination of the female body. With that in mind:

Islam has also been concerned with procreation as it is indicated in many verses of the Koran (7:189-191; 31:10; 51:49) that consider procreation as the aim of coitus *(nikah)*.It is then, the love of having a child, based on the intent to procreate, that corresponds to the general purpose of the Muslim man, which is to worship Allah." (Al-Zubair 1991, p. 19)

Postscript
Convergences and Divergences

The significance of human sexuality

Anthropology and bioethics, as previously noted, are related by the concept of the human person. Sexuality is taken into consideration as a core component of the human being, who is a sexual being,. This justifies the relationship between anthropology and sexuality.

Sexuality Can only be Understood in an Anthropological Context

The Catholic Church and Islam refer to sacred scriptures as a basis for their respective stances and teachings about human sexuality. While the Catholic Church provides in her teachings a discourse on sexual ethics, Islam refers exclusively to the *Shari'a* which regulates all aspects of Muslim personal life (including sexuality), and addresses any moral conflicts that may arise. The role of the *Shari'a* is so important that it covers the field : it allows no space for anthropological thought which may depart from the *Shari'a*. Accordingly, the convergences and divergences between Catholicism and Islam relating to human sexuality complicate the task of an interreligious bioethics, for their anthropological ideas will always have fundamentally different bases, and produce different views.

Convergences

Both Catholicism and Islam agree that 'man' and thus humanity is a creation of God. This induces certain similarities regarding human sexuality between the two religions. These include:

1. According to both the Biblical and Koranic scriptures, sexuality does not stem from internal exigencies felt by the individual or societal obligations, but rather from the

will of God to create man and woman as sexual beings. Sexual being is thus fundamentally engrained in the created human nature of man and woman. Both the Bible and Koran assert that sexuality is a gift bestowed upon 'man' when created, and is characterised by beauty and goodness which are both attributes of God.

2. The Bible and Koran explain the purpose of creating two sexually distinct but complementary human beings, as beings who are orientated to procreation in order to ensure the continuance of the human species on earth. The Koran states: "marry such of you as are solitary ..." (24:32). Similarly the Bible asserts that humanity should "be fruitful, multiply..." (Gen 1:28). Accordingly, God grants to human beings power to transmit life through their sexuality.

3. Just as the doctrine of the Catholic Magisterium is based on the Bible, so the Islamic *Shari'a* is based on the Koran. Both provide teachings on sexuality which work from an essential and fundamental principle uniting sexuality and marriage: any sexual relationship outside of marriage is prohibited, thus making marriage the sole state in which sexuality find its purpose and its justification , and where the desire for sexual relations can be fulfilled . Accordingly, both Catholicism and Islam have made sexuality an integral component of man's fundamental vocation, and consider promiscuity, adultery and "free love" to be moral sins.

4. From the beginning, both man and woman were created as sexual beings, as asserted in both the Magisterium and *Shari'a*. Accordingly, the sexual act is itself sacred, and allows each person's femininity or masculinity to be expressed through their body. However, this does reduce corporeality to sexuality, for the body has other functions. The practice of single sexual acts does not express the totality of sexual life, and in the same way sexual life does

not express the entirety of human life, or fulfil the person as a whole. The manifestation of human sexual capabilities is neither the purpose nor meaning of human life.

5. Sexuality is a form of communication in which a person is able to express their connections with the world, others and themselves, as the Magisterium and *Shari'a* both confirm. The union of persons is, in effect, a way of shedding loneliness, enabling communication and developing bonds with others. Therefore, man and woman, being aware of their physical sexual difference, feel an attraction and are guided towards one another.

Divergences

Even though there exists commonality between Catholicism and Islam regarding sexuality, the divergences far outweigh the similarities. These include:

1. Catholicism views sexuality as a sacred power that has been bestowed by God on humanity for the good of man and woman, not excluding their pleasure, although its supreme but not sole gift is said to be the gift of children (*Gaudium et Spes* no. 50). Islam on the other hand, places greater importance on the pleasure of the flesh, which is in itself, the primary aim of satisfying sexual instincts (Bousquet, 1990).

2. The Bible presents the human being as a sexual being, who is in "the image of God" and his likeness. Thus, a dual sexual polarity of male/female is actualised in the image of God. The Koran, on the other hand, states that man was created as a sexual being by Allah, although he was not created in Allah's image, and therefore sexuality lacks a transcendental dimension.

3. Sexuality, according to the Bible, is a vocation of giving and receiving by "becoming one flesh." In the Koranic view, sexuality is limited to coitus *(nikah)* and is essentially a male activity.

4. Biblical references to sexual relations are expressed in terms of "knowledge" (Gen 4:1), that is, more than just the encounter of the male and female body. It is the communion between two people who learn to know and recognise one another. The Koran however, uses the term coitus *(nikah)* when referring to human sexuality. Coitus *(nikah)*, which has a significant place in the Koran, refers to sexuality in a one dimensional sense where there is no encounter of two persons, but is the physical expression of male virility and primacy through the sexual act.

5. The Bible states that man and woman are united when enacting sexual relations through the metaphor of *one flesh*. It is an act that is not exclusively for the purpose of procreation, yet it is presented as a gift: in love, man gives himself to the woman, and vice versa. In the Koran, on the other hand, "sexuality is certainly not reduced to procreation, but there is physical pleasure inherent to the being living it" (Bouhdiba 1986, p. 113). The sexual act then is first and foremost an act of pleasure particularly for the man, and subsequently something performed for procreation.

6. Biblically portrayed as an abiding in communion, sexuality is an act of equality between the man and woman. In this regard, God created woman as an interlocutor and equal companion for man, to help man emerge from his solitude. However, in the Koran overcoming solitude is only at the physical level, as sexuality involves a "bodily

presence, [which] is a call towards others on a carnal level" (Bouhdiba 1986, p.113). As such, the creation of woman was to provide man with an outlet or source of carnal pleasure, and not as an interlocutor and equal companion for man.

7. In the context of the covenant between God and 'man,' the Bible presents sexuality as an expression of love, denoting a reality that transcends sexuality, enabling both men and women to become part of the dynamic *agape*, that is the very nature of God. The Koran however presents sexuality in two aspects – procreation through the physical union between man and woman; and as coitus *(nikah)*, which is chiefly important as providing the Muslim man with sexual pleasures.

8. Chastity presents the major divergence between Catholicism and Islam. As confirmed in the Magisterium of the Catholic Church, chastity is a major virtue where consecrated persons choose, in the image of Christ, not to marry in anticipation of life in the Kingdom of Heaven. Accordingly, marriage is the proper state for physical sexuality, and remains an option or a life choice for the faithful. In Islam, the Koran the core belief is that Allah created everything in couples (51:49), as it is in the Bible. However, Muslims regard sexuality as a necessity, a right and a duty. Following the example of the Muslim Prophet, exercising sexuality becomes a pious obligation, and coitus *(nikah)* a universal law. The *Shari'a* does not accept any mortification of sexual instincts, which it considers to be an attack against life and God's will. Therefore, voluntary chastity and castration are blameworthy (Bouhdiba, 1986).

9. Although the Catholic Church and Islam agreed on sexuality within the state of marriage, there is a major difference. The Catholic Church regards marriage as a sacrament given to one man and one woman, and confines sexuality to within marriage for the purpose of procreation and for the good of the couple. Therefore, human sexuality is not objectified or reduced to being a pleasurable act, but it must be a significant and structural confirmation of the person (Pope John Paul II, 1985) which commands respect and acceptance. According to the personalist vision of Catholic bioethics, sexuality is a constitutive dimension of the person, and the Church recognises complementarity and dignified equality between spouses.

In Islam, the *Shari'a* refers to marriage as a contract *(keetab)*, between a man and a determined number of women. It is an act where man acquires, in a religiously permissible manner, authority over the female body. The Muslim man is permitted, by the *Shari'a*, to have four legitimate wives and an undefined number of concubines if he is able to support them (Bousquet, 1990). The *Shari'a* highlights the importance of sexuality for the continuance of the human species, and also asserts that the sexual instinct is a strong power given to man that requires satisfaction. The *Shari'a*, entitles the Muslim man to the pleasure and enjoyment of the sexual act. Therefore, the act of the flesh is a blessing from Allah, and polygamy and the rotation of women are almost mandatory and unavoidable concomitants of the sexual act . These are the characteristics of sexual ethics in Islam.

10. The Magisterium of the Catholic Church states that sexuality is a union and complete communion between a man and a woman which is based on equality and dignity. This is fulfilled through a sexual relationship that is justified by the free will of each to express their love in sexual relations; a love that is based on God's creative love, as manifested in Jesus Christ. On the other hand, and based on the Koran, the *Shari'a* links the practice of sexuality to the will of man, while the woman is subordinate to him. As such, the sexual relationship within Islam is not a union between two people, but rather between an active male party of man and his passive female partner who is considered to be a sexual organ and an object of pleasure and satisfaction for him (Ibrahim, 1994).

In Islam, the concept of love does not exist as such: love is merely related to sexuality, giving the recommendation of the Muslim Prophet that man must treat his wife well. Any idea of symbiosis between husband and wife – except for the idea of coitus *(nikah)* – seems absent from the *Shari'a*. Thus, coitus *(nikah)* is a sacred mission of the Muslim male which leads him to Allah, according to the Koran (Bouhdiba, 1986).

While the Islamic viewpoint of sexuality is so physical as to actually be opposed to the equality of make and female, certain Islamic scholars and authors nonetheless call for respect and equal rights for women. In this regard, Aroua (1990) states:

In the name of Allah and in the name of elementary justice, the woman must retrieve an active position within society, not only as a partner to man having the same rights as he does, but also as a citizen fully participating in the historical destiny of society, and finally, a supreme dignity, as a believer individually responsible before Allah for her acts, thoughts, body and soul. (p. 265)

In respect of the coming life, Islam teaches of materialistic pleasures in paradise, especially the unlimited sexual activities and other pleasures while the Catholic Church teaches that the Kingdom of God is not a place where, men and women are given and taken in marriage, but it is a place where there is only peace and joy in the presence of the Lord. (Matthew 22:30).

Finally, the Catholic perspective of sexuality is one that is both spiritualist and egalitarian. Sexuality is rooted in human nature, and marks both man and woman equally, without consuming them. Transcending their sexuality, the human person is enriched rather than weakened.

Part Three

The Significance of Human Corporeality

Introduction

For corporeal beings, coexistence is merely existing with or for others in this world. The corporeal dimension of 'man' has been reflected upon throughout the history of thought (Mercatali, 1985). Thus, when contemplating the anthropological foundations of bioethics, one cannot dismiss the corporeal reality of 'man. Trying to identify the anthropological foundation of bioethics, in both Catholicism and Islam, we will discuss the human body in terms of a purely philosophical anthropology. Accordingly, in this part, we shall attempt to reflect upon the concept and understanding of the human body, and to relate this concept to bioethics.

No one can deny that in today's society there exists a new outlook on the human body. It is obvious, and one can see clearly that each human body is unique. If someone were to ask who owns the human body, the spontaneous answer would be: "My body certainly belongs to me." Yet, in a religious context, the response might be: "My body belongs to God." To understand the basis of these answers , one must take into consideration the disparity between two different anthropological approaches, one which, emphasises the unity of 'man' without denying that the body belongs God, while the other also stresses the unity of the human being but confirms that the body belongs to the human person.

In this regard, the human body acquires its significance by belonging to a human person who assumes responsibility for it: it is not a question of anthropology, biology or philosophy. However, it is essential in bioethics to understand to whom the body belongs and to whom it is subject.

To respond to this question, we will discuss the human body in both Catholicism and Islam below, highlighting the similarities and differences between the two religions.

After presenting the corporeal reality of 'man' in Catholicism and Islam, Part Three will conclude by highlighting the similarities and differences between the two.

5

Bioethics and Corporeality in Catholicism

Catholic study of the human body has been s vast and ongoing: it will be impossible to fully explore it here. Accordingly, only the Biblical viewpoint and the contemporary teaching of the Magisterium will be examined. These disclose a view of the corporeal subject which differs from the contemporary secular vision of the human body, wherein it is considered to be an object, as opposed to a visible revelation of the human person. By virtue of understanding 'man's' "unitotality" – as discussed in the first part of this book – it is possible for the modern day Church to comprehend and evaluate the significance and actions of the body. The Bible and the teachings of the Church simply aim to inculcate respect for the visibility of the human being through the body, where 'man' is a relational subject created in the image of God.

The basis of Catholic bioethics is represented by the *personalist* approach. Sgreccia (1994) maintains that a personalist approach, anchored in ontology, is the basis for Catholic bioethics, and that this approach stems from the physico-spiritual unity of the human being. It is also based on the Thomistic vision of 'man,' which is the union between body and soul, where the spiritual soul captures two connatural abilities: to be oneself and to animate the body. This approach discloses how human activity is always a physico-spiritual unity, and it highlights how the body plays an essential role in this activity. It is in this sense, that the affirmation of Marcel (1951) "my own body does not exist on its own, for I am my body" can be understood.

The above affirmation contradicts every notion of the human body as an object; for, in the Catholic perspective, the ontological value of the body is manifested through its mediation and relationship with the world, society and history.

The body in the theological tradition of the Church

It is evident that the subject matter of the 'body' has a central place in the theological tradition of the Catholic Church. This discussion will briefly review the Biblical anthropology of corporeality, which forms the foundation of the teachings in Catholicism. That is, we shall consider veterotestamentary (Old Testament) anthropology and neotestamentary (New Testament) anthropology. The connection between the two is clear through the definition of 'man', being the union of body and spirit. It can be stated that the Biblical perspective allows 'man' to state, "I exist as long as I am my body."

The body in the anthropological vocabulary of the Old Testament

The Christian revelation treats the body from both an existential and an ontological perspective. The language used in the Old Testament to depict the body is very rich, utilising terms that present the corporeal dimension of the human being. The most widely used Hebrew expressions are *basar* or *leb / lebab* (Brown, 1992).

The use of the term *basar* refers to the human person in the corporeal state, and is mentioned over 270 times in the Old Testament. In the first instance, when referring to the human person, *basar* means *flesh,* namely, the totality of the body. But more precisely, *basar* refers to the integrated human being. This expression highlights the corporeal, creaturely and existentially precarious condition of the human being. It also indicates the material substance that forms the body: the body of the man being formed from the silt of the earth, and the body of the woman from the body of the man (Gen 2:21). To illustrate this, we can read in the Old Testament:

> "... my body longs for you..." (Ps 63:1)
>
> "All humanity is grass ..." (Is 40:6)
>
> "For Yahweh is indicting the nations, arraigning all humanity for judgement ..." (Jr 25:31)

The Old Testament defines 'man' as *basar* before himself, the human community and God. Before 'man' himself, the term *basar* brings to mind the limited and fragile condition of 'man' who is subject to suffering and death. Before the community, *basar* implies that every human being takes part in the human condition. Before God, *basar* highlights the dependence of 'man' on his Creator who gave him the vital breath that made 'man' exist, whereby

> If he were to recall his spirit, to concentrate his breath back in himself, all flesh would instantly perish and all people would return to dust. (Jb 34:14-15)

Rocchetta (1993) suggests that the term *basar* does not solely identify the visible form of the human being, but also points to the sheer reality of the existence of the human being. Thus 'man' does not only possess a body; 'man' *is* his body.

As a result of Hellenistic thought, which entered Judaism through the Greek Septuagint translation of the Bible, veterotestamentary language often portrayed a negative image of the body. In this manner, the Book of Ecclesiasticus depreciates the body as a source of passion (Sirach 23:16-18; 47:19). The Book of Wisdom also presents a distinction between the immortal soul and the perishable body (Wis 8:19-20; 15:8). Negative undertones are also found in Wis 9:15 which states that: "...a perishable body presses down the soul." These Biblical citations clearly state the priority of the spirit over the body, suggesting the presence of a pre-existing soul and a body that is susceptible to human nature, and the direct cause of wrongful acts and sins.

In the Old Testament, *basar* thus indicates the integrated 'man' incorporating his corporeal aspect, as it relates to the living body. It is worth noting that the term *basar* is not used when referring to a corpse. Furthermore, even if the word *basar* expresses the material dimension of the human being, the human being cannot be *basar* without God (Lys, 1967).

A further characteristic of Biblical language is that it is "quasi-systematically metonymic:, that is, it often allows one word or phrase to be substituted for another closely associated term. This is evident through the use of the term *leb / lebab*, that is heart. These terms are mentioned over 860 times in the Old Testament and refer to the centre of activity of 'man,' and his faculties of intelligence, thus indicating the totality of the human person capable of thinking and choosing freely. Thus, the heart of 'man' is not merely a bodily organ; it is an aspect of 'man' himself in his totality.

In Hebrew, *leb* is also the centre of emotion (1 S 2:1; 1:8 and Ps 13:5; 28:7) and feelings (1 S 16:17). It characterises the human person in both his emotive and sensual realities. The heart, or *leb*, is also considered to be the origin of evil, for human sin against the divine will of God is not initiated from the body but from the heart (Rocchetta, 1993).

Although in the Old Testament, humanity was called into a covenant, it is only in the New Testament that the promise of salvation of body and soul was fulfilled and achieved. Accordingly, the body is not an object for display through the arts, or for the enjoyment of life's pleasures, or the development of literature to sing its praises (except for the Song of Songs). Rather, the body must be prepared to receive salvation to fulfil the promise of God.

The body in the anthropological vocabulary of the New Testament
The anthropological vocabulary of the human body in the New Testament is characterised by the "movement of incarnation" through

which the "word of God was made flesh, born from a woman, born under the Law" (Demaison 1996, p. 22). In this regard, Demaison (1996) states that the incarnation is a movement, because being incarnated assumes a relocation of an entity that has now reached a new state of being. However, where human beings are concerned, the previous state is notional, because at no point in time did they lack a body. This reveals and creates a new way of being for the living person, speaking and acting through the living human body.

Christ is the first-born of all creatures visible and invisible: humans are created in Him, body and soul. He is also the first-born among the dead, to reconcile and give life to 'man' by the blood of His cross (Col 1:15-20). This salvation cannot take place outside the body. The Sermon on the Mount translates this into the language of action (Mt 5:3-11); it is not only acts of physical aggression, violence and transgression, which make murderers and adulterers. Insults and lustful glances are in their own way acts of brutality (Mt 5:21-28). Henceforth, in order to understand the action of salvation, we must translate all the signs used by Jesus Christ into our ordinary lives, for Jesus treated bodies which were suffering, possessed, terminally ill or already deceased. These signs thus announce and manifest salvation through human corporeality, although the two had never before been definitively linked (Demaison, 1996).

The thoughts of St Paul on the body are worthy of attention. Influenced by Greek philosophy, the Pauline anthropological vocabulary is marked by a contradiction between the spiritual and corporeal dimensions of the human body where 'man' in his totality, is left to make a choice. This choice is either according to the spirit *(pneuma)* or to the flesh *(sarx)*. The two most frequently used terms for the human body are *sarx* and *soma*.

Sarx refers to the flesh as a creation, and is characterised by its existence as a perishable, weak and mortal being, distanced from God, and disposed to sin because of wrongful ancestral acts. According to

St Paul, *sarx* refers to the person as a whole in his visible reality, and or more frequently in his fragility and morality (Rm 6:19; 2 Co 4:11) (Rocchetta, 1993. It does not merely indicate a part of the human person(Rom 2:28; Eph 2:11)).

St Paul maintains that *flesh* designates the obsolete condition of 'man' – unlike *body* which refers to the dignity of 'man.' St Paul likes to point out this contradiction between the flesh and spirit (Gal 5:17; 2:20 and Rom 8), and occasionally expresses a negative concept of the carnal being, for "...mere human nature cannot inherit the kingdom of God: what is perishable cannot inherit what is imperishable" (1 Cor 15:50). According to Mercatali (1993), this internal struggle of supremacy of the spirit over flesh and the soul over body that St Paul emphasises, does not inevitably entail a repudiation of the dignity of the body. In fact, its primary aim is to balance forces within a human being in order to harmoniously make up the person who God created, Christ saved, and is destined to final glorification.

This means that because of his state, living in sin and death, the human creature is not capable of reaching salvation alone. When St Paul speaks of this conflict, he does not imply two different modes of action within the human being, but rather an opposition that exists between the human being as guided by the power of the spirit, and as guided by human weakness derived from sin. In other words, there is opposition between the old and new 'man' and not between body and soul, for God does not condemn the *flesh*, but rather the sin (Rom 8:3). This is why St Paul spoke of the body as the "flesh of Christ" (Col 1:24), and St John declared that "what is born of the flesh is flesh" (John 3:6). This discourse is most prominent when Jesus promises His own *sarx* to be eaten and his blood to be drunk for eternal life, and for the salvation of the world (John 6:51-56) (Schweizer, 1965).

Thus, *soma* refers to 'man' in his solidarity with creation and the sinful human condition, while acknowledging the value of his being, because he was created by God and owes his existence to Him

(Robinson, 1962). In general, *soma* implies a very positive concept of the body. It is no longer the flesh (*sarx*) of passion, sin and death, but the body of the baptism to be offered to God (Rom 12:1), with the awareness that "[the body] is for the Lord, and the Lord is for the body" (1 Cor 6:14). The body of the faithful is the temple of God, and he is therefore invited to glorify God through his body (1 Cor 6:19-20). St Paul in his letter to the Philippians says that "...Christ will be glorified in my body, whether by my life or my death" (Phil 1:20).

Soma then, is not equivalent to *sarx*, but to *basar*, to 'man' in his entirety whether in the internal structure or visible form. Thereby, corporeality is the locus where salvation takes place from the moment Christ was born of a woman according to the flesh (Gal 4:4), when He saved us by offering His body and when, through His resurrection, He made us into His own body. Thus, the corporeality of humanity was renewed by the glorified Christ and by the power of the Spirit, to become living members of His body (1 Cor 6:15) (Rocchetta, 1993).

Robinson (1962) points out that,

> *Sarx* and *soma* nominate different aspects of the relationship between man and God: while *sarx* designates the man associated with the creation but separated from God, *soma* designates the man associated with the creation as made by God. (p. 45)

The personalised body and the Bible

In line with the explanations provided of certain anthropological terms concerning the body in the Bible, it is suggested that the body can be comprehended through the personalisation of 'man.' This is evidenced in the Bible where each relationship with the self, with the world, with God and with others, can only be expressed, established and realised through the corporeal existence of 'man.'

Furthermore, the use of an organ name in the Bible is not meant "to indicate a part of a man, but rather the man as a whole" (Lacroix

1992, p. 216). This is significant in two ways: first as a reflection of the unitary and global mode according to which the human being is considered as one and unified. Secondly, it gives place neither to a spiritualistic vision of the body, nor to a materialistic vision that reduces the human person to merely a body, wherein the spiritual reality and the relation to God is forgotten.

Considered as the unity of vital power in corporeal existence, the human being, through his body, is able to establish relationships with the created world, with others and with God to whom 'man' owes his being and capacity to act. The personalised body secures unity with the spiritual and corporeal dimensions, both of which belong to a unique person who totally expresses a reality created and called to salvation. In sum, the Biblical stance on the body is not driven by "the spirit-matter dualism, but by the creature-creator duality" (Lacroix 1992, p. 216).

The body according to the contemporary Magisterium
If "the Hebrew concept of personality is that of an animated body rather than an incarnated soul" (Robinson 1962, p. 27), then it values corporeality so that 'man' may fulfil his existence through his body. The Magisterium of the Church has developed its teachings of this Biblical concept. The human body, the visible person, is by definition a "body-of-gift." Sexuality, as previously described, is considered to be the dimension where the significance of the body as a "body-of-gift" is best exhibited. Yet the dignity of the body is only apparent in light of the truth, as something created by God then saved and glorified through Jesus Christ.

The body: the visible human person
The history of the creation of 'man' as told in the Book of Genesis, describes 'man' as the masterpiece of God, and as the plenitude and centre of the created universe. His corporeality is an indispensable

part of the marvellous order of the creation. Thus "human life is irreducibly both corporeal and spiritual" (*Pontifical Council for Health Pastoral Care 1995*, 39). Accordingly, the body is the real symbol of human being, and corporeality is the representative plenitude of the spiritual "I," called to encounter and communion.

Placing the human body in its rightful position and demonstrating its dignity as a manifestation of the person, *Donum Vitae* (Congregation for the Doctrine of Faith, 1987) affirms that:

> By virtue of its substantial union with a spiritual soul, the human body cannot be considered as a mere complex of tissues, organs and functions, nor can it be evaluated in the same way as the body of animals; rather it is a constitutive part of the person who manifests and expresses himself through it. (3)

In the body, the person's "I" has a consciousness of oneself, others and God. In *Educational Guidance in Human Love*, the Sacred Congregation for Catholic Education (1984) states that:

> ... the body reveals man, "expresses the person" and is therefore the first message of God to the same man and woman ... (22)

Human subjects can only perceive themselves in and through the body: the body is an image that is oriented towards fulfilment. The corporeal dimension may not be considered to be a part of the human form, but rather the person's way of being and thus an expressive and self-realising manifestation of that personal being (Rocchetta, 1993). Therefore, any intervention with the human body:

> ... affects not only the tissues, the organs and their functions but also involves the person himself on different levels. (Congregation for the Doctrine of Faith 1987, 3)

Therefore, the approach of *personalist* bioethics demands respect for the human person in his totality.

In order to further reinstate the value of the human body, Pope John Paul II validates the distinctiveness of the revelation of 'man' through his body in *Acta Apostolicae Sedis*, and states

> Each human person, in his absolutely unique singularity, is constituted not only by his spirit, but by his body as well. Thus, in the body and through the body, one touches the person himself in his concrete reality. (Acts and Documents of the Supreme Pontiffs 1984, 393)

Further, the visibility of the person through the body cannot be explained except through the body being a "symbol" (Guiraud, 1980). By its unifying role which leads to understanding and living the human spirit, the body warrants being called a symbol, insofar as:

> The ontological pairs that form the structure of anthropology are focused in it: interior and exterior, cognitive and affective, ego and other, nature and culture. There is nothing more unifying that the body of man. (Ide 1996, p. 193)

Another aspect of the visibility of the person through the body is that it acts as a mediator with the world and society. It is an indication of the capacity of the human person to reach fulfilment, as it has both personal and human significance. Thus:

> ... the body is an incarnation in space and time, individual differentiation, expression and culture, and a relationship with the world and society. (Sgreccia 1994, pp. 39-40)

For the dignity of 'man' to exist, it is essential to know the relational value of the body, because a negative relation with the body entails a negative relation with oneself and others. Rocchetta (1993) states:

> He who does not respect his own being in his body and spiritual-corporeal unity, will find it difficult to respect the corporeal state of others and the human habitat where they live. (p. 10)

The human body: a source of moral obligations

The role of the human body is not limited to the visibility of the person: it is also, in some respects, the foundation of moral personal relationships. Thus, corporeality becomes the revelation of the person and of their morality. In fact:

> ... the body, in its biological make-up and dynamic, is the foundation and source of moral accountability. What is and what happens biologically is not neutral. On the contrary, it has ethical relevance: it is the indicative/imperative for action. (Congregation for the Doctrine of Faith 1987, 3)

The notion of the body as a gift negates any liberty to freely dispose of the body or to transmit this authority to someone else. This concept primarily insists upon respect for the body, thus:

> The natural moral law expresses and lays down the purposes, rights and duties which are based upon the bodily and spiritual nature of the human person. Therefore this law cannot be thought of as simply a set of norms on the biological level; rather it must be defined as the rational order whereby man is called by the Creator to direct and regulate his life and actions and in particular to make use of his own body. (Congregation for the Doctrine of Faith 1987, 3)

The above moral truth is founded on the *Catechism of the Catholic Church*, where it is asserted that the body, and spirit, has a full part in the creation of 'man' who, is in the *image of God*. Further, corporeality is to be experienced as a gift from the creative act of God, and a place of experience and encounter with Him.

However, the human person as the unity of body and spirit, is a source of morality and ethics. Thus:

> One cannot prescind from the body and make the psyche the criterion and source of morality: subjective feelings and

> desires cannot replace or ignore objective corporal conditions.
> (Pontifical Council for Health Pastoral Care, 1995, 41)

The dignity of 'man' requires that the human body does not exclusively satisfy desires that are in opposition to the objective truth of life. Without separation and divisibility, the body and spirit participate in the dignity and the human value of the person, as body-subject and not body-object, and in this way they make the body inviolable.

To accentuate the severe consequences entailed by a behaviour objectifying the body with the intention of abusing it, *The Charter for Health Care Workers* (Pontifical Council for Health Pastoral Care, 1995) highlights a connection between the dignity of 'man' and the dignity of God. An offence against the dignity of the human body is therefore an offence against God, the Creator and Master of life, for:

> The body cannot be treated as a belonging. It cannot be dealt with as a thing or an object of which one is the owner and arbiter. Every abusive intervention on the body is an insult to the dignity of the person and thus to God who is its only and absolute Lord. (42)

Whoever encounters a body, does not only encounter a body of tissue, but a reality that is sacred in itself, and a reality that is enriched from the vitality of the God of life. This reality is a sign of the transcendental presence of the body, and it is also under the sign of God's blessing. Therefore, an encounter with the body must always be made with reverence.

In Catholic anthropology, the body cannot be considered externally as an object which is to be analysed and studied as though it were an organic and purely biological reality *(body-object)*. Rather, the body must be perceived as the visible actualisation of personal subjectivity, united and individual, as the body of a person with all the greatness of personal being *(body-lived)*. In effect, this is Christian personalism (Rocchetta, 1993). Every interference with the body, in either the medical or civil context, must therefore take this fundamental relation between the body and moral law into consideration.

The spousal significance of the body

The body is at the centre of the requirements of moral law because it is a sexual body. The spousal aspect of the human body finds the true meaning of corporeality in self-giving. This perspective of the human body is elaborated by Pope John Paul II (1980).

Firstly, it is explained that a powerful bond exists between the mystery of creation, a gift born from love, and the sacred principle of the existence of 'man' as both male and female. The truth about the body and of sex of man and woman is a simple and pure truth. This bond is then vital for communion between persons. When man first sets eyes on woman, he simply asserts the identity of both human beings, and refers to woman as being: "This one at last is bone of my bones and flesh of my flesh!" (Gen 2:23)

Pope John Paul II (1985) adds that:

> ... (of) the Yahwist text, one can only say that this "body" reveals the "living soul," which man became when God-Yahweh breathed life into him ... His solitude before all other living beings began in virtue of this act. Exactly through the depth of that original solitude, man now emerges in the dimension of reciprocal gift, the expression of which – by the very fact the expression of his existence as a person – is the human body in all the original truth of its masculinity and femininity. The body, which expresses femininity "for" masculinity and, vice versa, masculinity "for" femininity, manifest the reciprocity and the communion of persons. It expresses it through gift as the fundamental characteristic of personal existence. (p. 183)

This sacred state of being and existence of 'man' as male and female, relates to original innocence (prior to original sin). On this subject, Pope John Paul II (1985) affirms that the discovery of the spousal meaning of the body consists of 'man,' as male and female, is presented in the whole naked truth and reality of his body and sex, in complete liberty from every constraint of body and sex. Created in love, and being endowed with masculinity and femininity, both of them are nude because they enjoy the same freedom of gift. This freedom is at the core of the "spousal" meaning of the body. The human body, along with its masculinity and femininity seen through the mystery of creation, is not merely a source of fertility and procreation as in the natural order of things. The body holds its "spousal" meaning, that is a capacity to express love through which 'man' becomes a gift and through this gift, fulfils the meaning of being and existing (Pope John Paul II, 1985).

Accordingly, when expounding the meaning behind the significance and existence of 'man' as both male and female (Gen 2:23), the body is in fact a witness to the creation. It is an essential gift, and a witness to the bountiful love of God (Ide, 1996).

The commentary of Pope John Paul II (1985) on the verse that mentions the original nudity of man and woman – nudity that is in no way shameful (Gen 2:25) – confirms that the human body is a creative gift. Man, aware of the procreative ability of his own body and sex, becomes at the same time free from the constraints that his own body and sex may impose on him:

> ... that "both were naked, but did not feel shame," we indirectly touch its root, as it were, and directly already its fruits. Interiorly free from the constraint of their bodies and of sex, free with the freedom of the gift, man and woman *were able to enjoy the whole truth, the whole self-evidence of the human being*, just as God-Yahweh had revealed it to them in the mystery of creation. (p. 187)

As a result, the inner freedom of the gift is central to the original nudity. This gift allows man and woman to mutually meet as the Creator intended, each as oneself. Man internally receives the woman in her femininity, receiving her for herself as she was intended by the Creator. Reciprocally, woman receives man for himself in his masculinity as he was intended by the Creator. This is the revelation and the discovery of the "spousal" meaning of the body (Pope John Paul II, 1985).

In this context, we understand that the human body is internally orientated towards the "sincere gift" of the person, revealing masculinity and femininity in their physical aspect, as well as unveiling the value and beauty that exceeds the simple physical dimension of the human being. Thus, the "spousal" meaning of the body related to the masculinity-femininity of 'man' is made complete. On one hand, this meaning shows a particular capacity to express love that makes 'man' become a gift. On the other hand, this reality underlines the capacity and the profound potential of a true affirmation of the person. As a result:

> the other – the woman for the man and the man for the woman – is through the body someone willed by the Creator "for his own sake," that is someone unique and unrepeatable, someone chosen by eternal Love. (Pope John Paul II 1985, p. 188)

The revelation and the discovery of the "spousal" meaning of the body are an explanation of the original happiness of 'man.' Even though this meaning undertakes multiple deformations, its significance subsists and demands to be revealed in all its simplicity and purity. It manifests itself in all its truth for it is the sign of the image of God, the road from the mystery of creation that meets the mystery of the resurrection of the body (Rom 8) (Pope John Paul II, 1985).

In this manner, the body holds a "spousal" meaning, given that the 'man-person' can only find himself through self-giving. If Christ revealed to man and woman another mission that goes beyond their matrimonial vocation – namely that of renouncing marriage for the Kingdom of Heaven – Christ has, through this calling, made the truth of the human person explicit. If man and woman are capable of making the gift of their own self for the sake of the Kingdom of Heaven, this is proof that the exercise of freedom is possible within the human body, and that this body effectively has a true "spousal" meaning (Rocchetta, 1993).

The body as a scene of salvation: redeemed and glorified in Jesus Christ

Disfigured by original sin, the human body is redeemed by Christ's resurrected body and destined for the glorification of God. In this sense, the body becomes the scene of meeting between God and 'man.' The *Catechism of the Catholic Church* (1995) summarises this doctrine as follows:

> The human body shares in the dignity of "the image of God": it is a human body precisely because it is animated by a spiritual soul, and it is the whole human person that is intended to become, in the body of Christ, a temple of the Spirit ... (364)

This finds its explanation in the sacrament of the Eucharist, where the body of Christ imparts divine life to the human soul and body. None but God who made flesh, can come towards 'man' and heal him by reconciling him with his own flesh and with God. The relation between the body of the faithful and that of Christ – which allows man to enter the glory of God on the day of his resurrection – is expressed as follows:

> We become God by becoming 'children,' 'sons,' that is by partaking in the dialogue of Jesus and his Father and letting our dialogue with the Father infiltrate the flesh of our own

> daily life: "You shaped a body for me." Our salvation is in becoming Body of Christ, like Christ Himself: in accepting to be received everyday by Him, in relying everyday on Him, in offering our body everyday to be the scene of the Word. We become God by following his path: in a descending and ascending movement. (Ratzinger 1977, pp. 67-68)

The resurrection of Christ, origin and illustration of our resurrection, fulfils us following His example, body and soul. As Jesus Christ was revealed as the Son of God through His resurrection from the dead, this dogma exhibits the full dignity of the sons of God (Rom 8:29). The resurrection of the body results in an anthropological and theological Christian dogma that forms the touchstone of the vision of 'man:' if the body was promised the same eternity as the spirit, then both of them and only *together*, form a unique person. In fact, the resurrection of the flesh teaches that the body of 'man' will be resurrected at the end of time, at the final judgment , that it is a promised eternity, and that it inherits the same destiny as the immortal spirit. The *Catechism of the Catholic Church* (1995) states:

> Christ, "the first-born from the dead" (Col 1:18), is the principle of our own resurrection, even now by the justification of our souls, and one day by the new life he will impart to our bodies. (658)

In the perspective of the Parousia or the second coming of Christ, the dynamics of the act of redemption provide a true opportunity for the human state, and in particular, for the body to be glorified for:

> ... we are expecting a saviour, the Lord Jesus Christ, who will transfigure the wretched body of ours into the mould of his glorious body... (Phil. 3:20-21)

In Summary

The human body, as conceived by the Catholic Church, is a "given body." 'Man' is created body and soul in the image of God, who saves the body and soul equally (Compagnoni, 1990). The body, as 'word' that was made 'flesh,' furnishes to each being self-revelation through an invitation to live the gift of life in history along with others on a path toward the Absolute (Rocchetta, 1993). However, the transformation of the spiritual-corporeal person of the "I" to the "I" of spiritualised corporeality can only be made through the spirit of the resurrected Lord. Thus: "The spiritual "I" of man is also incarnated; it is a spiritual "I" in a body." (Rocchetta 1993, p. 9)

The human creature is fully spiritual and fully corporeal in mutual interaction without a possibility of separation between the two. In this manner, the animated body as a manifestation of the totality of the person and their value is that they are the locus of relationships with the universe and society. They witness to creation, highlighting its inviolability whether in the horizontal sense, that is the relationship with others, or in the vertical sense, that is, the relationship with God.

6

Bioethics and Corporeality in Islam

As seen in previous chapters, man in Islam is a union between soul and body (Gindi, 1976). This union between the material and spiritual element, a constitutive aspect of 'man,' does not imply the equality of these two elements. In general, Islam perceives the soul as the principle of existence and the body as a mere "envelope." Chebel (1999) defines the body as being "a given" that specifies us as a subject-object. It is our envelope, our flesh, our image as seen by others and our signature" (p. 17). In an aim to explain this reality, Mahmoud (1989) states: "...with old age and weariness, the body becomes incapable of responding to the needs of the soul" (p. 77). This however, does not entail that Islam has a negative view on the body. In fact, Mahmoud (1989) adds that "...the perception of the body as a source of impurity and sin is not Islamic, but is opposed to Islam" (pp. 80-81).

The relationship between Islamic bioethics and corporeality is non-existent outside a context in which the body connects man to the world and the soul gives the body the ability to act, as well as placing within its reach the significance that it continuously transcends man's own earthly experiences. According to Chebel (1987), "this is why corporeality can only be fundamentally specific for each one of us" (p. 205).

The reality of the human body, expressed in this way in the Islamic tradition, as well in the contemporary *Shari'a*. Islamic thought regarding the body, is based on several texts, mainly the Koran and those various *Hadith* which frequently substantiate it.

The body in the Islamic theological tradition

In the Islamic theological tradition, the corporeal reality of man is directly related to the soul. The latter "commands the body and controls it. It is not its appendix" (Mahmoud 1977, p. 29). Consequently, the entire value of the body stems from the soul. It descends on the body to animate it and make it into a living being and leaves the body at the time of death, so that it can be transformed to dust (*turab*) once more. This view is based on the anthropological vocabulary of the Koran.

The body in the anthropological vocabulary of the Koran

The term "body", *gasad* or *gism*, is absent from the Koran. Nevertheless, the Koran implicitly refers to the human body in the context of creation and procreation. The Koran represents the body as the form that is most adapted to the existence of man. In this context, it can be observed that using an organ of the body in order to specify the body as a whole, the visible man may be a common feature of the Bible and the Koran. In fact, the term heart (*qalb*) is used frequently in the Koran. Generally, three expressions that enunciate the term "heart", as it is understood in the Semitic tradition are:

1. *Qalb* (plural *qulub*): meaning "heart", which appears 131 times in the Koran
2. *Sadr* (plural *sudur*): meaning "chest" and thus "heart", which appears 43 times
3. *Fu'ad* (plural *af'ida*): meaning "viscera" or "entrails", implying "heart", which appears 16 times.

The Islamic tradition considers the heart to be an organ of intellectual faculties: memory, attention, intelligence and wisdom. It is also the site of passion, sentiment, will and faith (Chebel, 1995).

According to Arnaldez (1971), the Koran presents numerous verses regarding the physical reality of man. God "created man of patter's clay" (15:26). Important are verses 23:12-14 where the concept of embryogenesis is found. The raw material of the human body is "the wet earth" with additional elements added successively – the *noutfa* that is fixed in the uterus, the *alaqa*, the *mudga*. From here, differentiation between bodily tissues takes place, that is bones and flesh. Then a "second creation" occurs containing the different phases of development from birth until death.

The development of the human body in the Koran is completed through a "second creation" that has particular significance. In fact verse 23:14, "Then fashioned We the drop ... produced it as another creation" (23:14) indicates that the body was given its definitive form and function, for:

> Allah made man a living being when he was inert matter: talking, when he was silent, and hearing, when he was deaf, seeing when he was blind. (Arnaldez 1971, p. 1296)

Allah has put inside and outside of him, in all his members and parts, a marvellous nature and admirable wisdom that cannot be adequately described.

The importance of the human body in the Koran is also shown by a verse that describes the direct intervention of Allah in its creation and formation: "He it is Who hath created for you ears and eyes and hearts" (23:78). Additionally, the Koran says of the physical reality of man that: "We created man of the best stature" (95:4).

According to a well-known Islamic scholar, Al-Razi (864-930 A.D.), verse 95:4 alludes to the exterior form and the balanced shape and form of man. Other commentators state that man is the only animal whose face is not directed towards the ground, but rather stands erect and uses his hands to pick up food (Arnaldez, 1971).

Moreover, in commenting on this same verse Al-Naggar (1996) asserts that the body of man was created as an integral and harmonious ensemble, with the intent of realising the purpose of his creation. If man was created to be the vicar of Allah on earth to fulfil his orders, his body must be the ultimate form of all, given that the human body gains value through its supreme end.

The body personalised in the Koran

The personalisation of certain body parts is observed in the Koran, in particular verse 24:24 with the tongues, hands and feet *(shama'il)*. Their role is to bear witness or proof:

> Till, when they reach it [the Fire], their ears and their eyes and their skins testify against them as to what they used to do.
>
> And they say unto their skins: Why testify ye against us? They say: Allah hath given us speech ... (41:20-21)

Further to the above, according to verse 17:36 on judgement day or the Day of Reckoning, questions will be asked about the acts of hearing, sight and of the heart *(fu'ad)*.

The corporeal dimension of being is revisited in the *Hadith* reported by Al-Bukhari (1984) in the context of symbolism linked to faith, that seems to take inspiration from the Koran and accentuate the role of the heart in the behaviour of the person. That is:

> There is a morsel of flesh that exists in the body; if this morsel of flesh is healthy, the entire body is healthy; if it is sick, the entire body is corrupted, right? Well, this morsel of flesh is the heart." (Al-Nawawi 1992, p. 34)

The above image of the impenitent heart is a metaphor for the faithful, good and bad.

According to the following Koranic verses, Allah fortifies and strengthens hearts:

> Who have believed and whose hearts have rest in the remembrance of Allah. Verily in the remembrance of Allah do hearts find rest! (13:28); and

> ... He hath written faith upon their hearts and hath strengthened them with a Spirit ... (58:22)

Further:

> Say (O Muhammad, to mankind) ... For he it is who hath revealed (this Scripture) to thy heart by Allah's leave, confirming that which was (revealed) before it ... (2:97); and
>
> Lo! therein verily is a reminder for him who hath a heart, or giveth ear with full intelligence. (50:37)

Masson (1976) presents various Koranic verses which outline the implied significance of the heart. Paradise is promised to the pure of heart. Conversely, the heart, ears and eyes of unbelievers are blind (22:46). Allah is all knowing, and knows what is in man's heart (33:51). Along these lines, the Koran warns believers against weaknesses of the heart which may be influenced by guilty desires (33:32). Some hearts are filled with doubt about Allah and the Last Day (9:45).

In this perspective, a *Hadith* describes a relation between Allah and his servant where the body is personalised through the different organs. Al-Nawawi (1992) states:

> My servant will not cease trying to be closer to Me through subrogation until he obtains My love, and when I will love him, I will be the ear through which he will hear, the gaze through which he will see, the hand with which he will grasp, the foot with which he will walk. If he seeks Me, I will certainly grant him My favour, if he beseeches my protection, I will certainly concede. (p. 106)

In short, it cannot be said that in the Islamic theological tradition, man is his body. Influenced by Aristotelian philosophy, traditional and even current Islamic thought leans towards the identification of man with the soul. This is substantiated in the Koran, where it states: "the Spirit is by command of my Lord" (17:85). Arnaldez (1971) refers to Al-Razi providing the following commentary:

We know by necessary intuition that the spirit is what man refers to when he says: "I". But what is this "I"? The organic body? However, none is oblivious to the fact that its parts change and are constantly replaced. If man is not this body, is he a body that exists inside the organism? It cannot be one where the earthly element is dominant, for it would be bones, flesh, fat, tendons, and no one identifies man with these tissues that are "thick, heavy and gloomy." Neither can it be a body where the liquid element is dominant, for it would be one of the four liquids, and man is none of them. However, some think that blood would be an exception here for its loss begets death. This doctrine, writes Al-Razi, is strong and sublime and must be given thought for it is exactly relevant to the accounts of the divine books on the state of life and death". (pp. 1270-1271)

The body according to the contemporary *Shari'a*

If the purpose of human existence is to be with others, and being open to others, then this is only possible through the body and its language. The body is a presence before others, a memorial synthesis of the past, present and future before others and before society. It bears the possibility of mutual acquaintance and communion between men. This is how the contemporary *Shari'a* perceives the human body.

Some Islamic writers focus on the body in all its gestures, from smiles to tears and from gazes to the demeanor of the face. The body is the principle and sign of individual differentiation (Chebel, 1999). According to the *Shari'a*, the body can be viewed in four aspects. Firstly, the subject body is defined as the manifested person, and then as a source of moral requirements. From there, a discussion follows about the feminine body and the resurrection of the body.

The body and the visible person

The *Shari'a* is not reluctant to assert that the body is the person's visibility as intended by Allah. When the Koran speaks of the creation of "man of the best stature" (95:4), it indicates the physiological structure experienced as a manifestation of his spiritual structure.

In order to demonstrate the importance of relations between man and his body, Arnaldez (1971) basing himself on the theory of Ikhwan Al-Safa, a group of Arab philosophers of the tenth or eleventh century A.D., asserts:

> The term "man" is applied to this body shaped as a built residence and this soul that inhabits this body: these are the two parts of man; he is their sum, the reunion of the two. But one of the two parts is more noble; it gives the body its completion and thus attains perfection ("kamal"). The body is for the soul what the workshop is for the craftsman. (p. 1270)

Al-Naggar (1996) highlights that the body, through which the person expresses himself, is his medium to the outside world. Consequently and through the biological-spiritual aspect, man is endowed with intelligence and attains comprehension and culture.

Yet, the strong Aristotelian influence in Islam leads certain authors to state that the body does not represent the person. Mahmoud (1977) for instance states:

> If I am identified by my body, then how is it possible for me to dominate and subjugate it?...the simple internal control over the members of the body and over every instinct is the obvious proof of the superior and transcendent element that forms the human Me. (p. 29)

For this reason, the person is identified by his soul rather than the body, because the body remains an object while the soul is a subject.

The presence of the human person in the body also establishes a relation with the world. Referring to the Islamic tradition, Chebel

(1987) describes the human body as a "well furnished" residence, where:

> The soul being its householder, alongside its family and servants (the faculties). The head represents a high chamber, the neck an arcade, the throat a vestibule; the teeth are railings; the lungs symbolise a summer room and the heart, thanks to the energy that passes through it, the winter room. The abdomen is compared to a harem; the intestines are its place of leisure. As for the anus and urethra, they are the sewers. (p. 118)

Accordingly, each part of the body possesses an architectural, social, customary, military and geomantic function.

To conclude, it can be said that the concept of the body, as visibility of the person, is not very pronounced in the *Shari'a*. Some refer to the body as "the being of the expressive" because man is essentially "a corporeal presence, a being of the corporeal... From the outset, he seems as a hyphen between Ego, Alter and their immediate surroundings" (Chebel 1999, pp. 204-205).

The body as a basis of moral obligations

Yasin (1996) using the *Shari'a* and *Fiqh*, speaks of the relation between law and human body. He asserts that the legal scholars *(al-ulama)* divide the rights on the human body into two major parts: the rights of Allah on one hand, and the rights of the Islamic faithful *(al-abd)* on the other. The right of Allah is the law that insures the common good of the Islamic community, whilst the right of the faithful is for their own personal good.

Many of the *fiqh* recommendations note the right of Allah over the living human body (Yasin, 1996), for instance:

1. The prohibition of suicide, which is one of the major sins *(al-kabair)* (4:33). A *Hadith* is quoted that prohibits

suicide and affirms that whoever commits it will be condemned to the fire of hell for all eternity, for he who commits self-murder violates the right of Allah.

2. The prohibition of suicide is added to that of self-harm. In fact, it is outlawed for anyone to cut an organ from their own body or injure themselves for no reason, because a person does not possess an absolute right over their own body and organs.

3. An assassin must be punished, even when the victim's family forgives him. This right is enjoined by certain traditional schools of *fiqh* like the *Malikites* and *Chafi'ites*, for while the family's pardon satisfies the right of the believer *(al-abd)*, it does not satisfy the demands of Allah or the community.

4. The prohibition of alcoholic beverages is worth noting, given that alcohol impedes a person's reasoning. This means that sane reasoning results is a duty to Allah.

5. Finally, the rights of the community over the body of the individual are crucial. The exercise of this right results in the unity of the Islamic community and fraternity among the believers; this solidarity is to exist in time of happiness and sadness. As proof, Yasin (1996) refers to a *Hadith* stating:

   One faithful is for another faithful, one building that must remain erect ... The faithful are one body. If one organ is ill, the whole body becomes ill, suffering fever and insomnia ... The faithful wishes for his brother what he wishes for his own self." (p. 151)

Further, the *fiqh* contains many examples of the rights of the faithful *(al-abd)* over their body. Yasin (1996) presents the following:

1. Punishment for whoever assaults another person, injuring their organs. The same violence or assault must be inflicted upon the offender. However, if the victim or the victim's family forgives the offender, the offender will not be punished, although he is obliged to reimburse them. Nonetheless, given that Allah's rights are inviolable, punishment is necessarily meted out when the *Shari'a* is scrupulously applied.
2. According to the law professors *(fuqaha)*, the aggression is not criminal where the victim has accepted or willed the violence. In fact, if one says to another, before witnesses: "Kill me", or "Cut my hand or my leg" and the other obeys, the offender is to be exempted from any punishment.

There is clearly a connection between the right of Allah and that of the faithful *(al-abd)* where the body is concerned. The true right of Allah over the human body is that it should accomplish good throughout the body of the faithful, and that the community might profit from that. Hence each organ of each individual of the community rightfully belongs to that community and must serve, within its means, the good of that community. The healthy human body enables him to fulfil whatever the Most High demands of him, that is, the good of the community where he dwells, and prayer, charity, pilgrimage, and "effort", among many others.

Alternatively, the right of the faithful *(al-abd)* over their body remains personal. There is an obligation to subjugate it for the realisation of earthly well-being (such as shelter, food, and so on) and to prepare it for the final end, where the person shall receive reward or punishment. Yasin (1996) addresses the question of rights concerning the body of a deceased, other than the rights to burial and prayer, which apply to every Muslim. Legal scholars take two different stances on relevant issues. One stance maintains the right of the family of the deceased to manage the body, especially in the case of organ transplant, while the other rejects any form of transplant unless specified by the deceased in a testament. Yasin (1996) supports the latter stance.

In Islam, interference with the human body is regulated by the *Shari'a*. Hmida (1998) states that:

> The doctor and the surgeon, when interfering with the human body, meddle with the rights of Allah as well as the individual. Accordingly, they are urged not to harm the individual, otherwise they would be transgressing his right as well as Allah's right without his authorisation." (p. 177)

The human body may only be interfered with in conformity with the law. Abd Al-Qadir (1990) confirms this, while insisting on the respect of the human body. It is believed that man has no right to change the form or structure of their body, as it goes against human dignity and honour. Quoting a *Hadith* about the prohibition of any kind of interference with the human body, Abd Al-Qadir (1990) concludes that the Islamic *Shari'a* disallows the disposal of the human body or its organs, even after death, for the body does not belong to man but to Allah only.

Abu Al-Fadl (1995) states that in Islam all that man has and possesses was given entrusted to him *(amana)* by Allah, and so the *Shari'a* insists upon the sacred character of the human body. The human body is an *amana* and thus sacred. The teachings of the Koran affirm that Allah has honoured man and as man belongs to Allah, his body also belongs to Allah. Abu Al-Fadl (1995) adds that this is also applicable in the context of organ transplantation. Additionally, Nachabeh (1996) asserts that the law professors *(fuqaha)* agree on the concept that ownership of man's body is not equivalent to any other ownership, but it is an ownership of usage. This entails that man may only dispose of it for a major good. Similarly, Hatout (1991) states that:

> Allah endowed the body with respect and honour ... It must absolutely not suffer violence whether it is alive or dead...We do not possess our bodies, they are entrusted to us so that we may protect them, keep them alive and use them only however as permitted by the Creator. (pp. 103-117)

Islam therefore professes an absolute respect for the human body. No one completely possesses their body. The body is an *amana* for life, after which man is to report to Allah on the usage that he made of it. In Islam, the disposability of the human body is reserved for Allah and not to men as it is not their property.

The body of woman

The *Shari'a* gives lesser importance to women and requires that woman "completely obeys her husband except in what displeases Allah" (Boudjenoun 1996, p. 75). Whoever addresses Islamic anthropology is faced with a major problem in the status of woman and, in particular, the matter of the possession of her body. The question becomes: does the Islamic woman have rights over her own body?

Al-Rayyes (1995) suggests that it is evident that Islam has restores some dignity to woman by putting an end to the customs of some Arab tribes. These customs included killing or burning female newborns. It must also be recognised that Islam has established equality between man and woman in numerous domains such as education, science, and ownership (Djamila, 1997; Abdel-Wahab, 1994). Yet, Islam has also, in many quarters, maintained inequalities and even upheld the principle of superiority of man over woman. This superiority is based on a perceived natural fact, namely the priority given to man at the moment of creation. The woman is a minor because she does not physically resemble the man and her role in life is limited to sexual relations with her husband and to the education of the children.

Al-Rayyes (1995) adds that the woman's body in the Islamic context is under political-religious authority, because obedience to authority is obedience to Allah. In this way, cloaked in religious ideology, political authority defines and dominates women's bodies. The body will be condemned and thrown in the fires of hell if it is rebellious, but will be rewarded with the pleasures of paradise if obedient to the authority of Allah.

In addition to this universal exigency, the body of woman must be subjugated to another private authority. It is the possession of man, be it the husband, father or brother, or even, at times, the mother who can assume certain functions of men.

Thereby, the Islamic society submits the woman's body to extremely strict laws starting from childhood with the parents' exaggerated anxiety over the body of their daughter, namely that she retains her virginity until marriage.

Moreover, she is required to remain in the family household in order to maintain a good reputation. The architecture and decoration of a traditional Islamic home are designed to hide the body of the woman and confine her indoors. Accordingly, when visiting traditional Islamic homes, villages, towns and countries, one will encounter high walls, securely locked doors, multiple curtains and windows with an indoor view rather than a street view. In effect, the feminine body in the Islamic outlook exists only to be incarcerated within four walls at the service of the patriarchal society (Dialmy, 1995).

In sum, the body of the woman in Islamic society is subject to the authority of others, especially of males. It is subjected to cultural and historical customs, laws and influences. It remains a prisoner of family relationships while hiding behind veils and long clothing. It may even seem that the female's best chance of liberation is through madness or possession by evil spirits.

The resurrection of bodies

The resurrection of the body is an absolutely fundamental aspect of the Islamic faith. This dogma of faith is asserted in a verse of the Koran where the creation of man is pointed to as evidence: "O mankind! If ye are in doubt concerning the Resurrection, then lo! We have created you from dust" (22:5).

Nevertheless, it should be noted that the resurrection of the body in Islam is in no way related to the sin of Adam. Similar to the Book of Genesis, the Koran (7: 22) recounts at the beginning of creation the story of the sin of disobedience to the will of Allah. Contrary to the Book of Genesis, Adam does not dwell on his sin since it was almost immediately forgiven (7:23). However, as a consequence of this sin, man had to walk away from paradise. Talbi and Bucaille (1989) state that even though the woman had no implication in this sin, Allah ordered Adam and his wife to leave paradise. The Koran states in 7:24-25:

> He said: "Go down (from hence), one of you a foe unto the other. There will be for you on earth a habitation and provision for a while."
>
> He said: "There ye shall live, and there ye shall die, and thence shall ye be brought forth."

From the above, there are three noteworthy points. First, "go down" means to leave paradise. Then "a foe unto the other" explains aggressiveness between humans. Lastly, man must, hereafter, live and die on earth; however, he will re-enter the lost paradise at the end of his life.

In this context, the resurrection of the body is regarded as a return to paradise. Confirming the dogma of the resurrection of the body in Islam, a certain *Hadith* – usually quoted to define the *necessary* religious beliefs and thereby the conditions of validity of faith – states that:

> The Prophet said: man possesses faith only if he believes in four things: 1- if he testifies that there is no divinity but Allah; 2- that I am the messenger of Allah entrusted with teaching the truth; 3- if he believes in resurrection (*ba'ath*) after death; 4- if he believes in the divine decree for good and evil, for sweet and bitter. (Al-Bukhari 1984, p. 630)

Gardet (1967) underlines the teaching of an Islamic school of thought, the Asha'arite teachings, which refuses to see in the "corporeal return" a common aspect between the three religions: Judaism, Christianity and Islam. For instance, this school states that the prophets that came previously to Muhammad, including Jesus Christ, have only ever preached the "spiritual return," whilst the Islamic prophet was the one to reveal the dogma of Resurrection of Bodies.

Furthermore, the purpose behind the Resurrection of Bodies is the final judgment, that is, accountability. Man stands before God with his "debits" (wrongdoings against the divine law) and his "credits" (good actions and, principally, his faith). The "debits" and the "credits" are assessed by the just Judge and, according to the result, the person will be either rewarded or punished (Chaltut, 1997). The resurrected body of the Islamic faithful will enter paradise where delights are foremost defined by sensual and corporeal pleasures.

In Summary

To conclude, it can be said that the Koran values the body because Allah himself created it. Even though the female body is regarded differently to that of man, and even confined to his guardianship, Islam perceives the human body as being created in the best of forms for it to be able to realise its purpose. The body must live up to a certain norm so as to embrace Islam and believe in Allah and his prophet. Therefore, it is put in the service of religion so that corporeality may fully take part in the act of faith. Corporeality is the visible part of the said faith. In this way, man according to Islam remains the privileged creature through his body that was directly made by the hands of Allah.

In this context, a *Hadith* of the Muslim Prophet provides confirmation of this vision of the body in Islam, whereby Muslims are required to take care of their body. It states:

Do not do so: fast then break your fast, stand up then sleep. You have duties towards your body; you have duties towards your eyes; you have duties towards your wife; you have duties towards your visitors. (Al-Bukhari 1984, p. 630)

Postscript

Convergences and Divergences

The bioetical foundations of Christianity and Islam

In interreligious bioethics, corporeality cannot acquire its full value without the spiritual dimension of the human person. The body is not a "possession," it is the visible expression of 'man.' It is evident in interreligious anthropology, that 'man' is not reduced to his body but is called to embrace and accept it in its limits and finite condition. The human body, the revelation of 'man,' has a unique significance in a theological or philosophical context. Accordingly, there exist numerous convergences and divergences between Catholicism and Islam.

Convergences

In Catholicism and Islam, corporeality is grounded in each of the respective Sacred Scriptures. Neither the Bible nor the Koran presents the human body outside of a direct relationship with the spirit, or a link with the world of the living. This anthropological reality is the foundation of the dignity of 'man' for interreligious bioethics.

Another common element – just as important as the former – is the concept of the body as a *body-of-gift*. The human body, created by God, does not belong to 'man' but to his Creator. Affirming this reality, neither the Magisterium nor the *Shari'a* authorise 'man' to dispose of his body as he pleases, but teaches him that his body is the subject of moral requirements. Protecting and defending the human body seems to be a second principle for interreligious bioethics.

Other convergences accentuate the common elements of the two anthropologies. The Bible and Koran concur that God himself intervened in creating 'man' and modelling his body. The Bible says:

"Yahweh God shaped man from the soil of the ground" (Gen 2:7). The Koran says: "Verily We created man of potter's clay of black mud altered" (15:26). In addition, both use the name of an organ to designate the entire body. In fact, the terms *leb* and *al-qalb*, that mean heart, are used by the Bible and the Koran to designate 'man' as a living body. The sacred texts along with the general Semitic tradition consider the heart as being the organ of intellectual faculties. It is also the scene of passions, feelings, will and faith.

Further, the Bible and Koran agree in frowning upon the hardhearted and incredulous. The Koran says: "Have they not travelled in the land, and have they hearts wherewith to feel and ears wherewith to hear? For indeed it is not the eyes that grow blind, but it is the hearts, which are within the bosoms that grow blind" (22:46). The Bible says: "Make this people's heart coarse, make their eyes dull, shut their eyes tight… use their heart to understand and change their ways and be healed" (Isa 6:10; Matt 13:15).

Moreover, the Magisterium and *Shari'a* agree on the sacred character of the body. As a revelation of 'man,' it is the true symbol of the human being. 'Man' is not reduced to his body, even though we attain the person in his concrete reality, in and through that body. In the last instance, the human body is a place of encounter and relationality. This relationality is *tri-dimensional* and is a connection with the world, society and God. The body as a medium remains the expression of the phenomenology of "I" in every gesture, from a smile to tears.

Divergences

Based on the preceding discussion in Part Two, there are two main divergences between Catholicism and Islam regarding their perception of the human body. The first is eschatological and relates to the resurrection of bodies; the second is anthropological and concerns the body of woman.

Even though Catholicism and Islam share a belief in the Resurrection of Bodies, they do not agree on the details or on the objective of the resurrection. In Catholicism, the resurrection of the body takes place only in Jesus Christ – a unique medium between humanity and God. Through his incarnation, death and resurrection, Jesus Christ saved 'man' and reconciled him with God after he was disfigured by Adam's sin. As maintained by Catholicism, the body is not the cause or origin of sin and evil. Yet, because of the indivisibility of its corporeal and spiritual aspects, the body sustained the repercussions of sin. In order to be saved, 'man' must then believe in Jesus Christ and unite with him in body and in spirit. Thus, the resurrection of the body takes place only in Jesus Christ who gives eternal life to those who believe in him. Life in the presence of God is the characteristic of this eternity.

Conversely, the Islamic concept of resurrection of bodies bears no relation to the sin of Adam. Unlike Catholicism, the sin of the first man was almost immediately forgiven by the Merciful Allah, and its sole consequence was the exclusion of Adam and his wife from paradise. The resurrection of the body on the Day of Judgment is, in fact, the return to the original paradise which is characterised by the different types of sensual pleasure promised to those who believe in the one Allah and his Prophet Muhammad.

The second of the main divergences between Catholicism and Islam concerns the corporeality of woman. According to the teachings of the Church, the human body is a body-of-gift. Whether it is male or female, it must be respected. Catholicism does not favour the body of a man at the expense of a woman, or vice versa. They are considered as equal in rights and human nature. This doctrine finds its basis in what is referred to as the "state of original innocence" of the human body prior to sin that disfigures everything. This state of simplicity, away from concupiscence of the flesh, reveals the "spousal" dimension of the human body. Along these lines, the present-day

Catholic Church teaches that the body is equally given to man and woman. It is entrusted to them and they will be held accountable for the way they handle it. Neither of the two holds more rights over the body than the other.

The vision of the female body is completely different in Islam. Woman was created for man and is therefore considered by the *Shari'a* to be subordinate to man, who is her superior. She is put under his protection, in both body and spirit. While the body of every Islamic man is subjugated to a political-religious authority and must be obedient to the rights of Allah and the community, the body of the woman, in addition to these two rights, is subjugated to the man. The woman's body is the possession of man, be it the husband, father or brother. She must be entirely at her husband's disposal to satisfy his sexual desires. Indeed if one was to ask the question "who owns the woman's body?" the answer in Islam would be that "it belongs to man rather than Allah."

Regarding the concept of the body in the Catholic Church and Islam, other divergences can be pointed out. They include:

> The Book of Genesis recounts the creation of the body of 'man' without specifying the different organs or mentioning the development of embryogenesis. However, the Koran not only recounts the creation of man, but also evokes an entire embryogenesis (23:12-19) and the creation of body organs: "He it is Who hath created for you ears and eyes and hearts" (23:78). These organs are personalised and act as witnesses to the Day of Judgment (41:19-21).

The Biblical vocabulary is richer than the Koranic vocabulary when it concerns the body. In the Bible, at least five expressions indicate the human body. They include two Hebrew terms: *basar* and *leb / lebab*, and three Greek terms: *sarx, soma* and *kardia* (*kardia* being equivalent to *basar* and *sarx*). However in the Koran, the expression "human body" does not exist as such. The only term that nominates the body is *al-qalb* (the heart) which is presented in several forms: *qalb, sadr and fu'ad* and, the plural *al-albab*.

The Magisterium of the Catholic Church strongly stresses the sacred character of the human body. It must not be considered as an external object of analysis or study, or merely an organic or purely biological reality. Rather it is to be considered as the temple of the Holy Spirit. Whoever approaches a body not only approaches a mass of tissues, but also a sacred reality in itself, a living manifestation of the God of Life. On the other hand, the sacredness of the human body is lacking in Islam. According to the *Shari'a*, nothing is sacred except for the spiritual, and in the case of man, his soul. This union or presence of Allah in the human body is inconceivable in Islam. Incarnation is a major point of divergence between Catholicism and Islam. The *Shari'a* insists upon the use of the body for the profit of the community from the perspective securing the accomplishment of man's mission as revealed in the Koran. That is, from the perspective of defining the role of corporeality.

These divergences in the concept of corporeality cast doubt upon the anthropological foundations of interreligious bioethics. Yet, we must acknowledge that the corporeal reality of man and woman is traced to the original creative act of God. In Catholicism, there is no separation and even less opposition, between the flesh drawn from the earth and life, between life and breath, or between breath and spirit. In Islam, man is the sole being in whom matter and spirit, body and soul, are united. Finally, human dignity leads to respect for the human body, which is an essential foundation for interreligious bioethics which is in turn necessary to minimise the risks of abusive interference with the human body.

Part Four

Health and Sickness: Ethical Principles

Introduction

As God's masterpiece in the universe, and endowed with life, 'man' has never been indifferent to the realities of sickness and health. On the contrary, 'man' has always been conscious of their great importance given that health and sickness are not merely matters affecting the physical organism, they are also relevant to his life aims. Medicine is involved in the corporeal state of any human being affected by the vicissitudes of life, such as the deterioration of health, recovery or death. Spinsanti (1990) speaks of administering medicine that is of relevance, for the human being must be at the forefront in the practice of medicine, with the person's importance being made obvious through the respect for personal1 suffering. In other words, administering *medicine* by the measure of man is the sole way of humanising it. Medical ethics are founded on morals and ideals, as well as on the religious and philosophical principles practiced in a given society. Consequently, it is not unusual to note that what holds an ethical value in one society may not in another. Depending on the norms of each community, the ethical attitude of an individual may be influenced by research, ideas and reflections, theologians, legislators, sociologists, economists, doctors, ethicists, and so on. The ethical debate is necessary in any given society, to establish standards of behaviour towards scientific and medical innovations.

The importance of health in anthropology cannot be overlooked. The connection between anthropology and bioethics calls for humanising medicine, an essential point in Catholicism and Islam.

Basing ourselves on the totality of this discussion thus far, Part

Four is also dedicated to the anthropological foundations of bioethics. Accordingly, ethical principles relating to health and sickness present a touchstone for every matter of bioethics.

The ethical viewpoint of health and sickness, in an interreligious perspective, is also relevant to our overall goals in this discussion. Through their religious teachings and their faith, Catholics and Muslims must distinguish between what is possible in medicine and the true good for 'man.' Thus emerges the major conflict between legal requirements and ethical duties, as legal affirmation does not entail moral validity (Serour, 1996).

Following the depiction of health and sickness in the theological traditions of Catholicism and Islam, the ethical principles of health care (more precisely autonomy, beneficence, non-malfeasance and justice) will be discussed. These principles, originating from the Anglo-Saxon context, will limit the scope of discussion when presenting the Catholic and Islamic points of view. As before, Part Four will conclude with a summary of the convergences and divergences.

7

Bioethics, Health and Sickness in Catholicism

In the teaching of the Catholic Church, life is a primary and fundamental good of the human person, insofar as *"Caring for life, then, expresses, first and foremost, a truly human activity in defence of physical life" (Pontifical* Council for Health Pastoral Care, 1995, 1). Every intervention in the domain of health is supposed to benefit life, as stated in *Charter for Health Care Workers* which asserts,

> ... health embraces all that pertains to prevention, diagnosis, treatment and rehabilitation for greater equilibrium and the physical, psychic and spiritual well-being of the person. (Pontifical Council for Health Pastoral Care, 1995, 9)

On the other hand, sickness is a reflection of the precariousness of the human condition. In his Apostolic Letter *Moto Proprio: Dolentium Hominum*, Pope John Paul II (1985) states that it is an experience that not only concerns the body, "but [affects] man in his entirety and in his somatic-spiritual unity" (2). The Catholic Church draws its concept of health and sickness from its theological tradition; the ethical principles of health care, addressed especially in the contemporary Magisterium, are a natural concretisation of this fact.

Health and sickness in the Catholic theological tradition

The tradition of the Catholic Church has bequeathed an extremely rich reflection on health and sickness. However, our discussion is limited to the research of foundations through Biblical revelation, for the Bible does not address the scientific aspect but, rather, exclusively addresses the religious significance of health, sickness and recovery in the design of salvation.

Health and sickness according to the Bible

The Biblical tradition widely addresses the issue of sickness. Correlated with recovery, sickness is among the principal Biblical themes. If health entails a full and vital power, sickness is primarily conceived as a state of weakness and deficiency (Ps 38:11). The natural causes of sickness are not probed. In fact, there are attempts to give religious explanations to calamities. Nonetheless, the concept of the Sacred Scriptures on this matter may be viewed through four major points:

1. Sickness and Divine Will

   The connection between divine will and sickness is very clear. When sickness strikes, God is the primary resort, for he is the master of life (Si 38:9-14). In this context, the *Catechism of the Catholic Church* declares that "the man of the Old Testament lives his sickness in the presence of God. It is before God that he laments his illness, and it is of God, Master of life and death, that he implores healing" (1502). It is Him who strikes and heals (Deut 32: 39). He is the doctor for man *par excellence* (Exod 15:26). Likewise, the sick approach those who represent him, the priests (Lev 13:49; 14:2) and prophets (1Kgs 14:1-13; 2 Kgs 4:21; 8:7). By humbly confessing their sins, they beseech the grace of recovery. The Psalter exhibits this by exposing their misery, imploring God for rescue, beseeching all his power and mercy (Ps 6:38; 41; 88). At times, healing comes in the form of a miracle (1Kgs 17:17-24; 2 Kgs 4:18-37; 5) (Giblet and Grelot, 1981).

   The New Testament does not provide a clear answer on the connection between sickness and divine will. Throughout His ministry, Jesus Christ encounters people stricken with illness. He does not interpret sickness through a narrow perspective of retribution (John 9:2), but rather sees it as an evil that makes human beings suffer as a result of sin. It is a sign of the power of Satan over 'men' (Luke 13:16). Jesus Christ feels compassion (Matt 20:34) which incites Him to act. He does not linger to distinguish natural illness from demonic possession, and "He drove out the spirits with a command and cured all who were sick" (Mt 8:16) (Giblet and Grelot, 1981).

2. The Connection between Sickness and Sin

   Sickness is no exception in a world where all depends on divine causality, and thus it is impossible not to interpret sickness as a punishment from God that strikes 'man' (Exod 4:6; Job 16:12; 19:21; Ps 39:11). Spontaneously, the religious sense of 'man' draws a connection between sickness and sin. The Biblical revelation does not contradict this, but merely specifies where this tight connection is to be seen. Since God has created 'man' to live, sickness and death are considered as an opposition to His profound intention. They are the consequences of original sin. In this perspective, there is a strict relationship between the ancestors' sinfulness and sickness. In this context, it is one of the signs of the wrath of God against a sinful world (Exod 9:1-12) (Giblet and Grelot, 1981).

   Yet, alongside this tradition is another trend of thought that underlines how illness may also strike the just. The Old Testament only admits two types of answers. When illness strikes the just as in the Books of Job or Tobit, it may be a providential test to show their fidelity (Tob 12:13). In the case of the suffering just, the servant of

Yahweh, sickness may sometimes constitute atonement for the sins of sinners (Isa 53:4).

3. Healing: Sign of the Advent of the Messianic Times

   The Book of Job is an excellent illustration of the second of the two above-mentioned lines of thought. In some cases in the Bible, sickness may be the consequence of personal sin. This is evident when Jesus Christ, after healing the paralysed man of Bethesda, tells him not to sin again (John 5:14). Alternatively, there is a hidden connection between sickness and the power of Satan. Jesus spent a great part of his public life healing the ill, driving out evil spirits and demons from the unwell (Mark 1:32-34; 3:7-11; Matt 4:23-24).

   Healing the sick and driving out demons are two forms of the same victory of Jesus Christ over sin. To the sick, Jesus Christ gave health for their body and spirit, liberating them from sin (Luke 5:18-20; John 5:14; 9:35-37). This position is a fundamental attestation of the coming of the Kingdom of Heaven among 'men' in Jesus Christ. At any rate, from the Biblical perspective, the healing of the sick remains the sign of Messianic times (Isa 53:4; Matt 11:4-6; Luke 7:21-23).

4. Paschal Mystery and Sickness

   If the son of God came to this world as the "doctor" of sinners (Mark 2:17) taking the infirmities of humanity upon himself (Matt 8:17), He has given them a new meaning. He has not eradicated sickness but, through suffering and sickness, He has given 'man' the possibility of partaking in the event of redemption. Similarly, the *Catechism of the Catholic Church* states: "By His passion and death on the cross Christ has given a new meaning to suffering: it can henceforth configure us to Him and unite us with His redemptive Passion" (1505). St Paul who repeatedly experienced illness (Gal 4:13; 2 Cor 1:8; 12:7-10) knows that sickness does unite 'man' to the suffering Christ, for:

... we carry with us in our body the death of Jesus so that the life of Jesus, too, may be visible in our body. (2 Cor 4:10)

However, the Book of Job does not clearly demonstrate the meaning of Job's trial. By contrast, however, the New Testament does indicate the meaning of suffering when it says that the believer rejoices because "...in my own body to make up all the hardships that still have to be undergone by Christ for the sake of his body, the Church" (Col 1:24). Sickness, suffering and death are thereby integral parts of salvation (Giblet and Grelot, 1981).

Through Jesus Christ, sickness is a path to redemption. It is a Paschal scene, in which 'man' must be prepared, whereby "Jesus has the power not only to heal, but also to forgive sins; he has come to heal the whole man, soul and body" (*CCC* 1503). When a baptised person lives their ailment as a moment of encounter with the Resurrected Lord, infirmity becomes a vocational situation that unifies the sick with the mystery of Christ's Redemption (Rocchetta, 1993). The miracles of healing performed by Jesus Christ anticipate, to a certain extent, the state of perfection that humanity will finally recover in the Kingdom of God, in accordance with the prophecies (Giblet and Grelot, 1981).

Health and sickness in the contemporary Magisterium of the Catholic Church

Health and sickness have always been two of the most worrisome problems for the human conscience. They have an explicit connection to the person as a whole. Christians are also familiar with the complexity of this problem. However enlightened by the Bible, they have an adequate and profound approach to the mystery of existence marked by the alternation between health and sickness.

The tradition of the Catholic Church follows the example of Jesus Christ and his Apostles who were not only interested in the spiritual well-being of the sick, but also their corporeal wellness. In keeping with this pattern, the current Magisterium of the Catholic Church insists upon the salvific dimension of suffering.

Health is a gift, sickness is a misfortune

For the Catholic Church, health is a precious gift from God. This fact is confirmed by the *Catechism of the Catholic Church* (1995) that states:

> Life and physical health are precious gifts entrusted to us by God. We must take reasonable care of them, taking into account the needs of others and the common good. (2288).

The health of 'man' is threatened by several factors that a healthy person is capable of avoiding. One can ruin their own health through work overstrain, taking drugs, such as alcohol or tobacco, or surrendering to carnal pleasures.

Gaudium et Spes (Vatican II, 1965) recommends not only conserving one's own health, but also not endangering that of others. In this perspective, the ethical dimension of life is deeply ingrained in the spirit and freedom of 'man.' Some illnesses and problems arise from wrong ethical choices (drugs, alcohol, HIV, violence, deprivation of goods necessary for health). To responsibly manage one's health is relevant to the balance of the person and is, in itself, a good for that person (Sgreccia, 1994).

Catholicism considers health to be a precious good that must be cultivated and protected. It is precious: however, it is not the highest value. Health must give 'man' the opportunity to assume his own responsibility towards God and towards his neighbour. Being in the service of God through consecrated life or in the service of others through civil professions (such as a doctor, nurse, politician or the like) does not entail the ability to recklessly put life at risk. Lack of care or disregard for health is not the only anti-human and non-Christian behaviour, so too is over-treatment which proves in reality to be pathological.

Conversely, sickness is a physical dysfunction and does not affect the person in their totality . It is primarily a manifestation of the weakness and finitude of the human being. In this way,

> Illness and suffering have always been among the gravest problems confronted in human life. In illness, man experiences his powerlessness, his limitations, and his finitude. Every illness can make us glimpse death. (*Catechism of the Catholic Church* 1995, 1500)

Sickness is more than a clinical fact that is medically controlled. It is the condition of a human being, the sick person (Pontifical Council for Health Pastoral Care, 1995). In this context, sickness has significance when it is lived in close union with the sufferings of Jesus. John Paul II (1985) asserts this reality in *Moto Proprio: Dolentium Hominum* while saying,

> Christ's redemption and his salvific grace reach the whole man in his human condition and therefore reach also illness, suffering and death. (2)

Thanks to this Christian vision, even though sickness entails suffering, it is not a misfortune but can be the occasion for a more serious Christian life. When faced with sickness, the person is called to adopt a triple salutary attitude towards it:

> ... an "awareness" of its reality "without minimising it or exaggerating it"; "acceptance", "not with a more or less blind resignation" but in the serene knowledge that "the Lord can and wishes to draw good from evil"; "the oblation", "made out of love for the Lord and one's brothers and sisters." (Pontifical Council for Health Pastoral Care 1995, 54)

The four ethical principles of health care and the Catholic Magisterium
The Magisterium has not made an official declaration of the four ethical principles of health care ethics: *autonomy, beneficence, non-malfeasance* and *justice*. Since the moment Catholicism abandoned the Hippocratic paternalism of medical ethics for *personalist* bioethics, its evaluation of these principles was facilitated. In fact, the intrinsic good of the person that refers to the analysis of characteristics innate to a person's existence, indicates that these principles can be considered as such. Nevertheless, they do not offer an explanation of what is considered to be the good of a person and the autonomy of an individual. In the Catholic perspective, the relationship between doctor and patient, and doctor and society, cannot solely have a horizontal dimension. The ultimate reference for all parties (doctor, patient, and society) must not be within them, rather it must transcend them (Sgreccia, 1994).

In this sense, it can be seen that a formulation of principles without ontological or anthropological foundations renders them sterile and vague. In the following, the four principles of health care ethics will be discussed, as viewed in the Catholic context.

1. Autonomy

    Respect for the person is a priority in all branches of Christianity, as all people are the children of God, created in his image. Faith in the life of the Holy Spirit (God personified) in each person calls for and reinforces this respect. However, current ideals of autonomy embody an unreal dream of self-sufficiency independent from God, the community, reason and reality that is unacceptable (Finnis and Fisher, 1993).

    Yet, in the health domain, the autonomy of the patient mandates respect for their rights. Hoose (1993) believes that each person in the medical profession must respect the patient's right for self-determination by providing them with sufficient information on their condition to decide the best treatment from those available.

Nonetheless, autonomy in a medical ethics context is often reduced to the two rights of the patient such as "privacy" and "free choice." The problem arises when, through these two patient rights, the principle of autonomy becomes a pretext to rationalising the termination of life of certain patients and the handicapped, that is, it becomes a pretext for the practice of voluntary euthanasia (Finnis and Fisher, 1993).

2. Beneficence

    The traditional purpose of a doctor's care is the promotion of patients' good health and treatment for their ailments. But in practice, this principle of beneficence involves another moral principle, that the end does not always justify the means. In this sense, beneficence encompasses the medical act in its totality. Thereby, true beneficence is not to be strictly focused on a given purpose, but must take into consideration the question of the means to reach that purpose and the intentions of practitioners (Finnis and Fisher, 1993).

3. Non-malfeasance

    Primum non nocere ('first do no harm') is classically the first principle of medical ethics according to the Hippocratic Oath. As pointed out by Finnis and Fisher (1993), three forms of malfeasance are common in health care practices: untruthfulness, murder and mutilation.

    Untruthfulness

    In medical practice, untruthfulness is to make patients (or their family) believe or accept something that goes against their own interest. Nevertheless, revealing the truth to a patient is a double-edged argument for bioethics: to disclose the entire truth or to not say anything at all can at times be destructive for the morale and health of the patient. However, lying remains harmful.

Murder

Even though it is a violation to the fundamental right to life given to every human being, concretely murder is of course an evil in medical practice. Whether in the form of abortion, euthanasia or assisted suicide, malfeasance remains an abominable practice and an intrinsically evil act.

Mutilation

Respect for the life of human persons includes respect for their physical, psychological and spiritual integrity. Non-malfeasance prohibits mutilation even where consent is granted, because it damages the fundamental good of the person (Finnis and Fisher, 1993).

Nonetheless, beneficence and non-malfeasance are not sufficient to guarantee the goodness of a medical act. Hoose (1993) restates the principle of double effect in a manner which he considers is practical and effective to guarantee the morality of medical intervention, so that:

"All our actions have more of an effect ... the evil effect may be justified if all four of the following conditions are fulfilled:

1. the act performed is good in itself.

2. the good effect does not result from the evil effect.

3. the person acting intends only the good effect.

4. there is a proportionate reason for causing the harm."
(Hoose p. 47)

4. Justice

The principle of justice refers to the mandatory equality in medical treatment according to the needs of each patient and especially for the poor and the marginalised. Since justice in the medical domain relates to society's commitment to realise the good of each person, it is joined to the principle of subsidiarity (Sgreccia, 1994). Moreover, given that justice respects all people and seeks their good, it includes the principles of autonomy, beneficence and non-malfeasance (Finnis and Fisher, 1993).

Finally, the Catholic Church sees the cause of the poor and the marginalised as one that is relevant to justice and an ethical value when it comes to health care. Along these lines, Hoose (1993) underlines the need for hospitalisation and care for a stranger who could otherwise be easily excluded, such as a person placed on a waiting list or one faced with a rejection and not being given medical care. That person however, is a member of humanity and with whom it is possible to develop a relationship. Perhaps in this case, this relationship is fundamental so that the customary practices in the medical world do not exclude anyone.

In Summary

Evidently, the Catholic Church perceives health as a gift from God, while sickness is a sign of the fragility of the human condition. The Fall, caused by original sin, is the only reason for sickness. Yet, God does not abandon 'man' in sickness; it is to Him that 'man' should turn to in an act of faith. The compassion of Jesus Christ towards the ill and his numerous acts of healing particularly marks the perception of sickness in the Catholic Church. Indeed, it is only through the salvific suffering of Jesus Christ that the suffering of 'man' acquires a meaning.

The unification of corporeal healing to the spiritual healing in the mission of Jesus Christ has initiated a new alliance with God. This alliance shows that the absolute value of life is not physical health, but the relation with God. Thereby:

> If morality requires respect for the life of the body, it does not make it an absolute value. It rejects a neo-pagan notion that tends to promote the cult of the body ... (Catechism of the Catholic Church 1995, 2289)

In this perspective, we come to understand the necessity and value that the Catholic Church tenders to each ethical principle in health care.

8

Bioethics, Health and Sickness in Islam

Islamic medicine is defined by ethics and deontology, in accordance with the prescriptions of the Koran and the divine *Shari'a* (Chiffoleau, 1997). Medical practice concerns the human being in a state of sickness. In this perspective, the maintenance of health is a point in common between anthropology and bioethics.

In general, the Islamic viewpoint on the issue of health is positive: health is considered to be the natural state of each human being in the world, whereas sickness is accidental and requires care (Abdul Hameed, 1981). According to Islamic anthropology, man in his corporeality can normally be in three states or modes of existence: health, sickness and a state that is neither proper health nor sickness, for instance being convalescent (Siouti, 1994). Historically, it seems that Islam highly values health and treatment of illnesses (Fazlur, 1984).

The following discussion will highlight the concept of health and sickness in the Islamic theological tradition, particularly in the Koran. Afterwards, the point of view of the *Shari'a* outlining the four ethical principles of health care will also be discussed.

Health and sickness in the Islamic theological tradition

The Islamic medical tradition is very rich. However, this discussion will principally cover only the Koranic teachings which ground the four ethical principles of health care.

Health and sickness according to the Koran

For Muslims, the Koran is the primary source for evaluating matters related to health and sickness. Even though few verses concern medicine or health care in a practical sense, the Koran is seen, in a practical sense, as "a healing and a mercy for believers" (17:82). In this sense, wellbeing and health are among the first blessings that Allah gives to man, for without health man cannot enjoy freedom of action nor accomplish his duties towards Allah or towards others. No other good is equal to health; it is a gift from Allah (Johnstone, 1982).

The importance of health in the Koran is evident in the various verses that speak of healing (41:44; 17:82). Yet the great Healer is Allah, the Creator who gives man the possibility to find a remedy. This is especially indicated in the verse: "There cometh forth from their bellies a drink diverse of hues, wherein is healing for mankind" (16:69). Nonetheless, turning to Allah in sickness seems to be an act of faith and trust: "...when I sicken, the He healeth me" (26:80). Conversely, the Koran ensures for the faithful a spiritual healing: "For those who believe it is a guidance and a healing; and as for those who disbelieve, there is a deafness in their ears, and it is blindness for them. Such are called to from afar" (41:44).

Consequently, sickness can be considered as punishment to those who do not believe in Allah and his Prophet. In fact, the Koran brings to the faithful spiritual and corporeal healing. Furthermore, this healing is related to the principle of divine determination, meaning that Allah can and will abolish sickness forever (Fazlur, 1984): "Naught of disaster befalleth in the earth or in yourselves but it is in a Book before We bring it into being" (57:22).

However, other texts of the Koran – and similarly in the Gospels – deny any relation between sickness and punishment from Allah: "No blame is there upon the blind nor any blame upon the lame nor any blame upon the sick nor on yourselves" (24:61; 48:17). The Koran offers spiritual remedies for corporeal afflictions: "And whoever among you is sick or hath an ailment of the head must pay a ransom of fasting or almsgiving or offering" (2:196).

Nevertheless, the body's health is inseparable from the tranquillity of the soul which is, in turn, closely correlated with the behaviour of man in life (Fazlur, 1984). Thereby, Islam calls upon man to set his life right in order to preserve the grace that is health: "That is because Allah never changeth the grace He hath bestowed on any people until they first change that which is in their hearts" (8:53). Health is thus praiseworthy, it is a gift from Allah, and sickness is at times inexplicable, but is not outside the divine will.

Finally, the Islamic theological tradition relates that the Prophet himself showed interest in medicine and concocted drugs. *The Medicine of the Prophet* (Siouti, 1994) holds a place of great importance and considerable value in the eyes of the Islamic faithful. Like the Koran, the *Hadith* confirms the effectiveness of prayer during sickness, as "prayer is healing! Healing for the soul and alleviation for physical sufferings" (Al-Bukhari, 1984).

Other *Hadith* speak of sickness and remedy saying:

> God did not send down sickness without sending down its remedy and whoever wants to learn this remedy learns it! and whoever wants to ignore it ignores it! (Al-Bukhari, 1984)

In terms of the importance of health, a *Hadith* reports that an Arab asked the Prophet: "After prayer, what am I to ask God?" Muhammad answered: "Ask for health" (Al-Bukhari, 1984). For Islam, it is evident that health has priority after the rites of worship, because "certainly no one has ever received anything more precious than health" (Falzur 1984, p. 590).

Health and sickness according to the contemporary Shari'a

Evidently, the contemporary *Shari'a* supports the Koranic vision of health and sickness. Health is shown as a gift and sickness is a misfortune. Islam encourages its devotees to seek treatment, for it is better to be treated than to patiently endure sickness (Seyyed, 1976). This context underlines the necessity of ethical principles for health care.

The gift of health and misfortune of sickness

In the times of the Prophet and according to Arab philosophy, health was in general the balance between the elements that form the world: temperature and the circulation of liquids in the human body. Conversely, sickness was the imbalance of these elements and the remedy was to restore this equilibrium, with the healer always being Allah. Al-Bar and Sibai (1993) assert that the *Shari'a* insists on treating the body well and conserving it in the best of conditions, because "your body has its rights on you" (Al-Bukhari, 1984).

Health is a gift from Allah whereas sickness is a source of suffering, grief and anxiety. A sick person experiences the suffering and fragility of their body as well as bearing anxiety in their soul. Islam is interested in the treatment of both. Since the inception of Islam, Islamic medicine has not separated the treatment of the body from that of the soul. From this, it is understandable that the *Shari'a* insists that the sick turn to the divine will above all (Al-Bar and Sibai, 1993).

On the other hand, while referring to the *Medicine of the Imams*, Falzur (1984) says that Shiites confer suffering and sickness with a meaning that does not exist entirely for the Sunnites, stating that

> This task, unlike that of the Sunnites, highlights in an unusual manner the spiritual merits of suffering and strongly advocates that the faithful must not consult a doctor before his illness has reached such an advanced stage that it surpasses tolerable suffering: "one night of suffering is more praiseworthy than an entire year of worship to Allah," adding that: "no one falls ill without having committed sin and sickness is purging ... In fact, you will be rewarded (in your sickness) for you have been resilient." (pp. 589-590)

In general, the Islamic religion urges the healthy to preserve their health and the sick to seek treatment and be hospitalised where necessary for recovery (Seyyed, 1976). Subsequently, the healthy man must strive to "enjoy (health), so as to remember it when he falls ill" and according to the Hadith, "take your health to your sickness" (Al-Bar and Sibai 1993, pp. 90-91).

In short, sickness according to the contemporary *Shari'a* is neither a punishment from Allah nor the wrath of the heavens, but it is still a misfortune. If a follower of Islam endures it with patience, it purifies the heart from sin (Hatib, 1985; Ferre, 1983). It is evident that illness is dreaded, an ordeal and a hardship for the Muslim, as it is at times incurable. It must then be accepted as the will of Allah, as man must render to the fact that he bears no importance in comparison to Allah's will. Thus, Allah alone can restore health to the ill (Athar, 1989).

The four ethical principles of health care and the contemporary Shari'a

The contemporary *Shari'a* has aligned its four ethical principles of health care with Islamic medical ethics. Serour (1996) claims that the *Shari'a* supports other principles such as the respect for human life and the protection of humans from any form of exploitation. Even though they have not all been applied since the dawn of Islam, they have been progressively established. Given that Islamic medical ethics follow Hippocratic morals, two of these principles have already been pointed out and taken into consideration: beneficence and non-malfeasance. In addition to the Hippocratic Oath being integrated into the education of Islamic doctors, Serour (1996) refers to Islamic bioethics and the work of Abil Hassan Ibn Radwan (998-1061 or 1067 A.D.) – an Egyptian scientist and doctor – who pointed out that the doctor must be characterised by seven virtues. Among these virtues, he included the three principles of beneficence, non-malfeasance and justice.

Hippocratic ethics is still relevant in today's Islam. The extraordinary progress of medicine and the complexity of medical problems require new medical ethics. However, the principle of autonomy, which is in contradiction with Hippocratic paternalism is the problematic point in Islam. For instance, the oath of new Egyptian doctors only includes the three principles: beneficence, non-malfeasance and justice (Serour, 1996).

A subsequent development has attempted to introduce the principle of autonomy but, it has remained "in principle." For example, autonomy was introduced in the oath of Islamic doctors and was adopted by the First International Conference on Islamic Medicine held in Kuwait (1981) and published by the Kuwait Medical Association in 1982. According to Serour (1996), the four ethical principles of health care are incorporated in this oath. First of all, it asserts that the doctor must respect the person's dignity and privacy and must not divulge their secrets (autonomy). Then, doctors must protect human life in all its stages whatever the circumstances and conditions, and must do their best to save it from death, sickness, suffering and anxiety (beneficence). Afterwards, doctors must be committed to research and knowledge for the good of humankind and not for its destruction (non-malfeasance). Finally, doctors must offer treatment to acquaintances and strangers, to the righteous and sinners, to friends and enemies (justice).

Thus perceived and presented, the four ethical principles of health care have recently been well-integrated into the medical oaths currently used in several Islamic countries. For example, the oath of the Islamic Medical Society of North America also mentions these four principles (Serour, 1996). It clearly points out that the medical profession is sacred because it is connected to the human mind, dignity and life that must be respected (autonomy). It also confirms that doctors will sacrifice their life for the service, love and mercy of humankind (beneficence). Doctors who conform to the directives of Islamic *Shari'a* will not kill or harm a human being (non-malfeasance). Doctors will offer medical treatment to the poor and rich, educated and illiterate, Muslim and non-Muslim, black and white (justice).

Below, each of the principles is elaborated to further explain the Islamic vision of the four ethical principles of health care:

1. Autonomy

    The principle of autonomy implies respect for the human person in the doctor-patient relationship. It also implies participation of patients in the medical decision, be they male or female. A patient maintains autonomy when given the freedom to accept or refuse therapy at any time. On one hand, Islam links this principle with the grand creation of man, endowed with free will and reason. Indeed:

    > ... each individual can only feel free and independent when he is solely dominated by the supreme Creator of the universe who confers him power. (Serour 1996, p. 79).

    On the other hand, Islam effectively adopts medical paternalism as a way of life, even though it is in contradiction with autonomy.

    Serour finds the foundation for the principle of autonomy of the human person in the Koranic verse that says, "We created man of the best stature" (95:4). While creating man, Allah left him a sign of respect and autonomy (14:32-33) which is freedom of decision. As such:

    > Even though Allah created the body and soul of humanity and subdued all of creation in his service – another important sign of respect for autonomy – he leaves to the human being the freedom to make his own decisions. He may help the person to reach the right decision, however, the definitive decision is left for the person himself to make. (Serour 1996, p. 79)

    To underline the principle of autonomy in Islam and its relation with medical ethics, Hasan (1996) also confirms that the autonomy-freedom relationship originated from Allah himself, stating:

> The Koran knows that the spirit of man is the divine spirit itself; if Allah is free, this essential attribute is shared by man, vicar of Allah on earth. This is why he possesses a freedom delegated to him. The first time Adam made use of his freedom was in disobedience. Freedom in itself cannot be an intrinsic value; it is however the essential condition, indispensable to reach each of life's intrinsic values. (p. 96)

Hasan (1996) touches on the relationship between autonomy and paternalism, contending that if autonomy is a principle, then paternalism is a way of life. Medical paternalism is then natural in an Islamic society ruled by a patriarchal system, where:

> Unlike autonomy, paternalism is not a limited principle. It is dependent on many variables, in particular on socio-economic systems. It may be considered as a way of life where the individual is dependant on the breadwinner, the feudal or religious authority, even on the state authority that controls finances... This has had considerable influences on life aspects. Thus, paternalism became a way of life. It is practised within the family. Therefore, it is the family's wishes that doctors apply paternalism. (Hasan 1996, pp.96-98)

Unlike western society where the principle of autonomy has been applied for years, it seems that Islam still adopts medical paternalism. In the doctor-patient relationship, the autonomy of the patient is non-existent because the patient must follow the doctor's opinion. Even though Islam insists upon autonomy and freedom for man, it seems that this doctrine is not applied in the medical domain. Indeed, paternalism applied by the doctor or the family is the optimal way to complete the treatment of a patient.

2. Beneficence

The term beneficence (*birr*), one of the pillars of the Message of Islam, has several meanings in the Koran. Its most relevant meaning in the health domain is *al-shif'a*, meaning to heal from a sickness. Hasan (1996) evokes one of Allah's many names, the Healer, which is not different from the Christian concept of God as the source of healing.

The Koran encourages good, and even orders it: "We hasten unto them with good things" (23:56). In Islam, individuals and communities are called to as good, so that they are rewarded with paradise (2:215; 3:104). Beneficence to the sick is a remedy to their ailments, and:

> There cometh forth from their bellies a drink diverse of hues, wherein is healing for mankind. Lo! herein is indeed a portent for people who reflect. (16:69).

In this verse, it seems as though beneficence must come from Allah to whoever is in need of it. In this perspective, Hasan (1996) speaks of doctors who invoke Allah for beneficence in their medical practice, and who:

> ... [do] not merely assume responsibility to heal the patient, but also resort to research and reflection. The traditional medical practitioner gives his prescription while invoking Allah to guarantee he is being beneficent to the patient. (p. 99)

The injunctions to perform good deeds in Islam are so wide-ranging as to even include the meeting of nations and people among themselves. A *Hadith* mentioned by Serour (1996) relates that Muhammad, speaking to Abu Zahr who was one of his companions, said:

> ... you must not depreciate a good action whatever it may be: even greeting your brother with a benevolent expression on your face counts. (pp. 81-82)

Islam recommends beneficence and endows it with great importance. In the medical context, the *Shari'a* presents the principle of beneficence as a necessity and encourages health professionals to work in the interest of the patient rather than their own. The doctor is prompted to respond to every call for help while considering it to be a religious duty. Thus, Islamic deontology and beneficence in medical practice can only be based on faith in Allah. Hasan (1996) also mentions the text on medical ethics by Ishaq ibn Ali al-Ruhawi, a ninth century physician. Al-Ruhawi speaks of the doctor's dignity whilst insisting that health is man's most precious possession. Thus, medical practitioners must be virtuous. Not everyone is qualified to practice medicine in the eyes of Allah, as this practice is solely reserved for those who possess a pure heart, have remarkable intelligence, love good and especially those who are merciful, and are compassionate and chaste.

3. Non-malfeasance

The two principles of beneficence and non-malfeasance are well set, not as an opinion but as an order from Allah to be obeyed by those faithful to Islam. In the Koran, Allah forbids the faithful to inflict harm:

> And there may spring from you a nation who invite to goodness, and enjoin right conduct and forbid indecency. Such are they who are successful. (3:104)

If beneficence is awarded in paradise, non-malfeasance is a commandment from Allah to be obeyed, under sanction of punishment: "And whoso doeth ill an atom's weight will see it then" (99:8).

Avoiding wrongdoing is a priority in the *Shari'a*. Islam rejects nihilism or minimalism in medical practice. In line with Hippocratic ethics, Islamic medical ethics adopts non-malfeasance as a basic principle. Even if at times this principle is used to put an end to life, the *Shari'a* nonetheless insists on saving life up until the last moment (Hasan, 1996).

According to the above, it seems that the two principles of beneficence and non-malfeasance are strictly related to moral rules. Doing good and avoiding evil, essentials in Islamic morals, are comprehensively applied to medical practice. For this reason, it is understood that these two principles are usually presented in Islam in a general manner. Perceived as part of the faith, beneficence and non-malfeasance imply the presence of God and as such, a *Hadith* declares that "God exists where good can be found" (Serour, 1996).

4. Justice

The ethical principle of justice in health care is acknowledged by the Islamic *Shari'a*. Even though the Koran does not speak of justice in this context, it formulates a principle whereby the *Shari'a* can adopt the principle of justice in biomedical ethics. In the Koran, Allah ordered the faithful to be equitable towards one another, for He dislikes the unjust: "For evil-doers there is no helper" (22:71). Justice is one of Allah's qualities, for He is "the Just" and His followers must imitate his justice (Serour, 1996).

The *Shari'a* emphasises several aspects of justice. It speaks, among other aspects, of familial, social, economic, individual and collective justice. The issue of justice in health care embraces all these aspects, namely social justice, individual and collective justice.

As presented by Hasan (1996), individual justice embraces three aspects that aim towards the respect of the human person, their rights, duties and aspirations. As to collective justice, it can be in the four following forms:

- Justice in social relations
- Justice in the application of the law
- Economic justice
- Politic justice

The principle of justice in health care is directly related to social justice. The matter of equality in access to health services is problematic in Islamic society. In fact, the majority of Islamic nations and people are in the Third World where sanitary services are poorly developed and where social security does not provide adequate hospitalisation. In this sense, Islam emphasises justice and equality while supporting the case of the oppressed and marginalised, especially every helpless sick person.

Health care nowadays is extremely expensive. It is thus problematic in developing countries. The monetary value and quality of health care casts a shadow over the implementation of the principle of justice in these countries. According to the *Shari'a*, justice denotes the availability of care and therapy for each and every person, even for those who do not possess the financial means to afford health care. A system based on value for money for health care in a poor society does not allow access to hospitalisation for the majority and is, consequently, an unjust system. In the health field, justice is an equitable service provided to everyone, and one of the major preoccupations of Islam is to ensure this justice is assured (Hasan, 1996).

In Summary

From the above discussion, it emerges that the matter of health and sickness in Islam is closely related to faith and divine will. This does not entail rejecting treatment, as Islam encourages medicine and health care. In this context, divine will merely means an Islamic doctrine stipulating that, in creation, there is no sickness without remedy. Indeed health is a gift, whereas sickness is a misfortune.

However, the four principles of ethical health care seem to be incompatible with a society adopting medical paternalism. Even though no problem is encountered where justice, beneficence and non-malfeasance is concerned, complications occur where autonomy is to be applied. Islam has its own outlook on freedom and autonomy. The reintroduction of paternalist medical ethics into post-modern medical society seems difficult, even impossible. According to Hasan (1996), the reason behind this is that the medical system in Islamic society is not on an equal footing with its equivalent in western societies where these principles originated.

Postscript
Convergences and Divergences

Health and sickness: ethical principles

The challenge of bioethics is related to health and sickness. The perception of 'man,' his vital integrity, the body, and its sane or morbid functionality, raises numerous ethical positions. This study, relating anthropology to bioethics is important because, when addressed in an interreligious context, it further clarifies the ethical debate. Hence there are convergences and divergences between Catholicism and Islam where the perception of health and sickness is concerned. Nevertheless, health care has always required ethical principles to regulate medical intervention and doctor-patient relations. Catholicism and Islam converge on certain ethical aspects of medical intervention and doctor-patient relations, but are in disagreement on others.

Convergences

The Biblical and Koranic scriptures do not provide a scientific definition of health or sickness. Nevertheless, they clearly underline their presence in the life of 'man.' Health is a blessing from God; sickness is a sign of human fragility. In times of sickness, 'man' must resort first of all to God; healing ought not to be merely physical, but should somehow deepen faith. Healing comes from God for He is the master of life and death.

The Bible and Koran both often consider sickness to be a punishment from God, and in the Semitic tradition, everything depends on divine causality. Therefore, the connection is made at times in the Bible (Deut 32:39; Hos 6:1) and the Koran (57:22) between sickness and God's retribution. However, it is necessary to point to texts that deny any connection between sickness and divine punishment in the Bible (John 9:3) as well as in the Koran (24:61).

Given that health is a gift from God, the Magisterium and the *Shari'a* recommend caring for it, for 'prevention is better than cure.' They affirm that nutritional and sexual abuse, wrong ethical choices such as drugs, alcohol, violence and deprivation of goods necessary for health bring damage to it. On the other hand, wellbeing allows 'man' to assume his own responsibility towards God, the community and his fellow human beings.

Health care is not to take place without ethical principles. The Magisterium and *Shari'a* are both in agreement over the principles of beneficence, non-malfeasance and justice. These three principles delegated with ensuring treatment for all, concern health care workers and social responsibility, and are naturally integrated in their manifestos of medical ethics.

Divergences

Three principal divergences between Catholicism and Islam can be pointed out concerning health and sickness. The first is on the subject of causality of sickness, the second on the meaning of sickness and suffering, and the third concerns the concept of autonomy as a health care ethical principle.

In the Bible and the Magisterium, the religious sense of 'man' draws a connection between sickness and sin. The former was only introduced to the world as a result of original sin. Healing may then be solely perceived as a grace from God who primarily demands repentance from the sinner. On the other hand and while not mentioning this connection between sickness and sin, the Koran and *Shari'a* state that everything, including both sickness and healing, is dependent upon the divine will of Allah.

In Catholicism, sickness and suffering hold a double meaning.

They are firstly a providential trial destined to prove the loyalty of the faithful in God. There is an abundance of examples in the Books of Job and Tobit, for instance. Sickness and suffering have a salvific aspect. To remove infirmities and illnesses, Jesus Christ took them upon himself (Matt 8:17; Isa 53:4) and gave them meaning by living them in His passion and resurrection. Suffering and sickness are no longer deprived of significance; they become an occasion to live in union with the suffering of Jesus Christ. According to Catholicism, the righteous who endure their sufferings thus prove their faithfulness to God and partake in the Redemption of Jesus Christ.

Alternatively, suffering and sickness in Islam generally lacks a salvific dimension, but rather has a purifying purpose. By calling the sick to prayer and fasting, the Koran confirms the connection between sickness and sin and thereby invites the Muslim to purify themselves, for "…whoever among you is sick or hath an ailment of the head must pay a ransom of fasting or almsgiving or offering" (2:196). As for the problem of the sufferings of the just, these remain unfathomable.

The third major divergence between the Catholicism and Islam concerns the principle of autonomy in health care. Catholicism chooses a health care system that is based on the patient's consent to therapy after disclosure from the doctor to the patient. Thus, autonomy is the patient's free choice of a treatment proposed by health professionals. Conversely, by adopting therapeutic paternalism, Islam confers doctors with the power to decide the treatment for their patients. As a result, even without considering the situation where a male doctor treats a female patient, the woman's autonomy has little scope, for the make doctor will often make the decisions for the female patient.

Given the unity of the human being, sickness does not remain a physical handicap but rather touches 'man' in his totality as a somatic and spiritual unity. The Magisterium points out that 'man', when struck by sickness, experiences his limits and finitude. For this reason, it recommends care for the sick and attention for the frail. Nonetheless, Catholic morals do not perceive this is as an absolute value and the Magisterium condemns abuse in treatment of health. However, as Islam perceives it, sickness does not strike man as a whole, but is rather limited to his physical dimension. Moreover, as sickness and suffering are devoid of meaning in Islam, a patient must seek health at all costs. The latter is only second to prayer in the scale of Islamic values. Nevertheless, the *Shari'a* speaks of illness as source of suffering for the body and anxiety for the soul and it inspires true fear.

Conclusion

Interreligious bioethics stands at the intersection of various religious ethical principles. The anthropological foundation of bioethics is centred on 'man' as the favoured creature of God. However, it is still unclear whether or not anthropology has the same states as an autonomous discipline within both Christianity and Islam. Anthropology affords a basis for applied ethics. This raises the question: can Islam, without an autonomous anthropology, formulate a discourse of moral theology and ethics, similar to that developed in the Catholic Church?

From this study, it has become apparent that Islam does not admit the independence of anthropology, theology, law, politics, economics and other like discourses which regulate human society. In Islam, all these areas are discussed as different aspects of the single Islamic *Shari'a*. Ethics and moral theology within the *Shari'a* are presented as rules and codes, rather than values and principles. Therefore, Islamic bioethics remains a regulatory discourse governed by the traditional values and teachings of the *Shari'a*.

On the other hand, over the past few centuries, moral theology and ethics in the Catholic Church has been considered a scientific discipline, enjoying its own intellectual autonomy. As such, there is no equivalent in the Islamic context. When discussing ethics, Islam has an unchanging viewpoint which is grounded in history and tradition, and dominated by the *Shari'a*. The Catholic Church however, continuously develops and evolves its teachings in ethics and bioethics.

An exhaustive reflection upon interreligious bioethics would not stop here. After examining issues of *general bioethics* in this discussion, the groundwork for my future dissertation into *specialist bioethics* has been laid and will be presented in a forthcoming volume of this series. The respect and dignity of the human person throughout each stage of the life cycle will be discussed – from conception, to old age, to death. In particular, matters such as in vitro fertilisation (IVF), human cloning, the termination of pregnancy, medically assisted deaths and euthanasia, organ donation, and the donation of gametes and embryos, will be incorporated in the interreligious discussion of *specialist bioethics*.

An interreligious approach to bioethics opens the gate for new dialogue between religions, in this instance Catholicism and Islam, and sets new prospects of mutual understanding within a multi-faith society. The anthropological foundation of interreligious bioethics is too vast to be explored in one study. This study is in itself a stepping stone in the expansive debate, dialogue and reflection of ethical issues that are addressed by the Catholic Church and Islam.

Bibliography

Abbud, A. A. 1978, *Al-insān fil-islām wal-insān al-mu'āsir (L'homme dans l'Islam et l'homme contemporain)*, Dar Al-Fikr Al-Arabi, Cairo.

Abd Al-Qāder, C. A. M. 1990, Magallat magma' al-fiqh al-Islāmi, Munaddamat al-mu'tamar al-Islāmi, vol. 3, no. 6, pp. 1761-1782.

Abd Al-Rahman, A., 1978, *al-Qur'ān was qadāyā al-insān (Le Coran et les problems de l'homme)*, Dar al-Ilm lil-malayin, Beirut.

Abdel-Wahab, A. 1994, *La Situation de la femme dans le Judaïsm le Chrustianisme et l'Islam*, AIEF, Paris.

Abdul Hameed, M. 1981, 'Medical Ethics in Islam', in *Studies in History of Medicine*, vol. 5, no. 2, pp. 133-159.

Abu Al-Fadl, M. E. 1995, 'Organ transplantation: Contemporary Sunni Muslim legal and ethica; perspectives', in *Bioethics*, vol. 9, no. 3-4, pp. 291-302.

Abu-Sahlieh, S. 1994, *Les Musulmans face aux droits de l'homme: Religion et droit et politique. Étude et documents*, Winkler, Germany.

Acts and Documents of the Supreme Pontiffs, 1984, 'Acta Apostolicae Sedis,' *Vatican Gazette*, no. 76, Holy See, Rome.

Al-Bar, M. A. and Sibā'ī, Z. A. 1993, *At-Tabīb, adabuh za fiqhuh (Le médecin sa morale et son fiqh)*, al-Dar Al-Šāmīya, Beirut.

Al-Bar, M. A. 1995, *Halq al-insān baina at-tubb wal-Qur'ān (La creation de l'homme entre la medicine et le Coran)*, Al-Dar Al-Sa'ūdīyalin-nasr wat-taūzī', Saudi Arabia.

Al-Bukhari, 1984, *Les traditions islamiques*, Maisonneuve, Paris.

Al-Buti, M. S. R. 1992, *Manhag al-hadāra al-insānīya (Method of the Human Civilisation in the Koran)*, Dar Al-Fikr, Damascus.

Al-Naggar, A.A. 1996, *Mabda' al-insān (Le principe de l'homme)*, Dar Al-Zaītūna, Rabat.

Al-Naggar, A.A. 1996, *Qīmat al-insān (La valeur de l'homme)*, Dar Al-Zaītūna, Rabat.

Al-Nawawi,. 1992, *Les quarante Hadith (no. 6)*, International Islamic Federation of Student Organisations, Kuwait.

Al-Qaradhawi, Y. 1973, *Al-Imān wal-hayāt (La foi et la vie)*, Maktabat Wihab, Beirut.

Al-Qaradhawi, Y. 1994, *Al-Halāl wal-harām fil-Islām (Le licite et l'illicite dans l'Islam)*, Al-Maktab al-Islami, Beirut.

Al-Rayyes, H. 1995, *Gasad al-mar'a, min sultat al-ins ila sultat al-gān (Le corps de la femme, de l'autorité de l'humain à l'autorite des fees)*, Sīna lin-našir, Cairo.

Al-Ša'ār, M. M. 1990, *Al-Alāqāt al-ginsīya fil-Islām (Les rapports sexuels en Islam)*, Dar al-Nafā'is, Beirut.

Al-Zubair, Y. A. 1991, *Maūqif al-Charī'a al-Islāmīya min tanzīm al-nasl (La position de al-Charī'a Musulmane en ce qui concerne la regulation des naissances)*, Dar al-Gīl, Beirut.

Aqqad, M. A. 1973, *Al-Insān fil-Qur'ān (L'homme dans le Coran)*, Dar Al-Salām, Cairo.

Arnaldez, R. 1971, 'Khalk (Création)', in *Encyclopédie de l'Islam*, vol. 2, pp. 1012-1020.

Arnaldez, R. 1971, 'Insān'', in *Encyclopédie de l'Islam*, vol. 2, pp. 269-1271.

Aroua, M. 1990, *l'Islam et la morale des sexes*, Office des Publications Universitaires, Algeria.

Assaf, M. A. 1991, *Al-Halāl wal-harām fil-Islām (Le licite et l'illicite dans l'Islam)*, Dar Ihya' 'ulūm al-din, Beirut.

Athar, S. 1989, 'Health guidelines from Quran and Sunnah', in S. Athar (ed.) *Islamic Medicine*, Pan-Islamic Publishing House, Pakistan, pp. 59-66.

Aubert, J-M. 1987, *Abrégé de la morale Catholique*, Desclée De Brouwer, Paris.

Autiero, A. 1990, 'Sessualità', in *Nuovo Dizionario di Teologia Morale*, Paoline, Milan.

Balic, S. 1991, *Dizionario comparator delle religioni monoteistiche. Ebraismo, Cristianesimo e Islam*, Piemme, Casale Monferrato.

Baz, P. 1992, 'Les Musulmans, leur corps, la maladie, la mort', in *Project*, vol. 23, pp. 60-74.

Bellino, F. 1997, *Antropologia e bioetica: Ricerca interdisciplinare sull'enigma uomo*, Massimo, Milan.

Borrmans, M. 1993, *Islam e Cristianesimo: Le vie del dialogo*, Paoline, Milan.

Borrmans, M. 1994, 'Islam et Famille', in *Se comprende*, vol. 94/11.

Boudjenoun, M. 1996, *Le Mariage en Islam: Modalités et finalités*, Maison d'Ennour, Paris.

Bouhdiba, A. 1986, *La sexualité en Islam*, Quadrige/ Presses Universitaires de France, Paris.

Bousquet, G. H. 1990, *L'Ethique sexuelle de l'Islam*, Desclée De Brouwer, Paris.

Brague, R. 1998, 'Islam et libre arbitre', in *Geopolitique*, vol. 61. Pp. 26-33.

Brown, P. 1992, *Il corpo e la societa: Uomini, donne e astinenza sessuale nel primo Cristinanesimo*, Einaudi, Torino.

Brugues, J-L. 1991, *Dictionnaire De Morale Catholique*, C.L.D, Chambray Lès Tours.

Catechism of The Catholic Church 1995, Libreria Editrice Vaticana, Holy See, Rome.

Chaltut, I. M. 1997, *Al-Islām 'aqīda wa Charī'a (l'Islam dogme et loi)*, al-Šurūq, Cairo.

Chebel, M. 1987, 'Visions du corps en Islam ou Corps, Corporel, Corporéité et Corporalité', in *Le cahiers de l'Orient*, vol. 8-9, pp. 203-226.

Chebel, M. 1995, *Dictionnaire des symbols musulmans: Rites, mystique et civilisation*, Albin Michel, Paris.

Chebel, M. 1999, *Le corps en Islam*, Press Universitaire de France, Paris.

Chiffoleau, S. 1997, *Médecins en Eygypte: Construction d'une identité professionnelle et project medical*, L'Harmattan, Paris.

Congregation For The Doctrine Of The Faith 1987, *Instruction On Respect For Human Life 'Donum Vitae'*, Holy See, Rome.

Colzani, G. 1988, *Antropologia teologia: L'uomo, paradosso e mistero (Corso di teologia sistematica)*, Edizioni Dehoniane Bologna, Bologna.

Compagnoni, F. 1990, 'Corpo e Vita', in *Nuovo Dizionario di Teologia Morale*, Paoline, Milan.

Demaison, M. 1996, 'Le corps à la lumiere de l'incarnation', Centre de Bioethique de l'Université Catholique de Lyon, 19 November 1996, Lyon-France.

Dialmy, A. 1995, *Logement, sexualité et Islam*, EDDIF, Morocco.

Djamila, D. A-M. 1994, 'Femmes et Islam en Occident', in *Encyclopédie Polotique et Historique des Femmes*, Presses Universitaires de France, Paris, pp. 771-785.

Durable, A.M. 1960, 'Foi en la creation et sentiment de creature dans l'Ancien testament', in *Lumière et Vie*, vol. 48, pp. 21-42.

Durand, G. 1977, *Sexualité et foi, Synthèse de théologie morale*, Cerf, Paris.

Fahd, T. 1959, *La naissance du monde selon l'Islam*, Seuil, Paris.

Faggioni M. P. 1995, 'La vita fra natura e artificio', in *Studia Moralia*, vol. 33, pp. 333-375.

Faggioni, M. P. 1995, 'L'uomo è ancora signore del creato? Tracce di etica ambientale', in *Antonianum*, vol. 70, no. 3-4, pp. 429-472.

Fazlur, R. 1984, 'Islam and Medicine: A General Overview', in *Perspectives in Biology and Medicine*, vol. 24, no. 4, pp. 585-597.

Fazlur, R. 1987, *Health and medicine in the Islamic tradition: Change and Identity*, Crossroad, New York.

Ferre, A. 1983, *Il problema del male e della soffrenza nell'Islam*, Piemme, Bologna.

Finnis J. and Fisher, A. 1993, 'Theology and the four Principles: A Roman Catholic View I', in G. Raanan (ed.), *Principles of Health Care Ethics*, John Wiley and Sons, New York.

Fisichella, R (ed.) 1993, *Commento teologico al Catechismo della Chisea Cattolica*, Piemme, Casale Monferrato.

Franck, B. 1980, *Famille marriage sexualité, dans une perspective chrétienne:*

Documents dy Synode Commun des dioceses Allemands (1971-1975), Beauchesne, Paris.

Frattallone, R. 1994, 'Persona,' in L. Salvino and P. Salvatore (eds), *Dizionario di bio*etica, Edizioni Dehoniane Bologna-Instituto Siciliano di Bioetica, Bologna.

Furlan, M. 1994, 'Etica Professionale,' in L. Salvino and P. Salvatore (eds), *Dizionario di bio*etica, Edizioni Dehoniane Bologna-Instituto Siciliano di Bioetica, Bologna.

Gardet, L. 1967, *Dieu et la destine de l'Homme*, J. Vrin, Paris.

Gardet, L. 1967, *L'Islam Religion et Communauté*, Desclée De Brouwer, Paris.

Gardet, L. and Arkoun, M. 1978, *L'Islam Hier-Demain*, Buchet / Castel, Paris.

Gelin, A. 1968, *L'Homme selon la Bible*, Cerf, Paris.

Giblet, J. And Grelot, P. 1981, 'Maladie et Guérison', in *Vocabulaire de Théologie Biblique*, Cerf, Paris, pp. 698-702.

Gilbert, M. 1974, 'Soyez féconds et multipliez', in *Nouvelle Revue Théologique*, vol. 10, pp. 724-742.

Gilbert, M. 1977, 'Une aide que lui corresponde. L'exégèse de Gn 2:18-24 dans les écrits de l'AT, du judaisme et du NT', *in Nouvelle Revue Théologique*, vol. 7, pp. 329-352.

Gindi, A. 1976, *Mu'allimat al-Islām (l'Institutrice de l'Islam)*, Al-Maktab al-Islāmi, Beirut.

Guiraud, P. 1980, 'Que sais'je', in *Le language du corps*, no. 1850, pp. 49-70.

Grelot, P. 1973, *Homme qui es-tu? Les onze premiers chapitres de la Genèse*, Cahiers Evangile, Paris.

Hachem, N. 1999, *La creation dans le Coran*, Doctorate in Philosophy, University Paris-Sorbonne, Paris.

Häring, B. 1989, *Liberi e fedeli in Cristo: Teologia morale per preti e laici-2*, Paoline, Milan.

Hasan, Z. 1996, 'Islam and the Four Principles: A Pakastani View', in G. Raanan (ed.), *Principles of Health Care Ethics*, John Wiley and Sons, New York.

Hatīb, H. I. 1985, *Al-wagīz fil-tūbb al-Islāmī (l'Abrégé de la medicine Islamique)*, Dar Al-Arqām, Jordan.

Hatout, H. 1991, 'Islamic consepts and bioethics', in B. A. Brody (ed.) *Bioethics Yearbook Vol. 1: Theological developments in bioethics 1989-1990*, Kluwer Academic Publishers, Boston-London, pp. 103-117.

Hmida, E. 1998, 'Ethique médicale. Universalité et culture', in *Le Courrier du Geri*, vol. 1, no. 2, http://stehly.chez-alice.fr/nouvelle6.html.

Hoeffner, J. 1973, 'La morale sexuelle à la lumiere de la foi. Dix questions et dix réspomses', in *Documentation Catholique*, no. 1682.

Hoose, B. 1993, 'Theology and the four Principles: A Roman Catholic View II', in G. Raanan (ed.), *Principles of Health Care Ethics*, John Wiley and Sons, New York.

Hottois, G. 1993, 'Déontologie et Éthique Médicales," in G. Hottois and M-H. Parizeau (eds.), *Les Mots de la Bioéthique: Un Vocabulaire Encyclopédique*, De Boeck-Wesmael, Bruxelles.

Ibn Qayyiem, A. 1974, *Raūdat al-muhibbīn wa nuzhat al-muštāqīn*, (Oasis of lovers and the promonade of seekers), Beirut.

Ibrahim, M. 1994, *Al-Gins fil-Qur'ān (Le sex dans le Coran)*, Beirut.

Ide, P. 1996, *Le corps à Coeur, Saint-Paul*, Versailles.

International Council of Churches Symposium 1974, *The vision of man in Islam, and the aspiration of man for peace*, Geneva.

John Paul II 1985, *Uomo e donna lo creó: Catechesi sull'amore umano*, Città Nuovo Editrice, Rome.

John Paul II 1979, Encyclical Letter '*Redemptor Hominis*,' Holy See, Rome.

John Paul II 1979, General Audience '*In the First Chapters of Genesis, Marriage Is One and Indissoluble*', Rome, http://www.vatican.va/holy_father/john_paul_ii/audiences/catechesis_genesis/documents/hf_jp-ii_aud_19791121_en.html.

John Paul II 1980, General Audience *The Human Person Becomes a Gift in the Freedom of Love*, Rome, http://www.vatican.va/holy_father/john_paul_ii/audiences/catechesis_genesis/documents/hf_jp-ii_aud_19800116_en.html.

John Paul II 1981, Apostolic Exhortation *Familiaris Consortio*, Holy See, Rome.

John Paul II 1983, 'Dangers of Genetic Manipulation', *Address to members of the World Medical Association*, Rome, http://www.ewtn.com/library/PAPALDOC/JP2GENMP.HTM.

John Paul II 1983, *Charter Of The Rights Of The Family*, Holy See, Rome.

John Paul II 1985, Apostolic Letter *Salvifici Doloris*, Holy See, Rome.

John Paul II 1985, Apostolic Letter *Motu Proprio: Dolentium Hominum*, Holy See, Rome.

John Paul II 1988, Apostolic Letter *Mulieris Dignitatem, On The Dignity And Vocation Of Women*, Holy See, Rome.

John Paul II 1991, Encyclical Letter *Centesimus Annus*, Holy See, Rome.

John Paul II 1993, Encyclical Letter *Veritatis Splendor*, Holy See, Rome.

John Paul II 1995, Encyclical Letter *Evangelium Vitae*, Libreria Editrice Vaticana, Holy See, Rome.

Johnstone, P. 1982, 'Medicine in Islam: A historical view', in *Encounter*, vol. 83.

Jomier, J. 1996, *Dieu et l'homme dans le Coran: L'aspect religieux de la nature humaine joint à l'obéissance au prophète de l'Islam*, Cerf, Paris.

Jonsson, G. A. 1988, *The Image of God: Genesis 1:26-28 in a Century of Old Testament*, Almqvist and Winksell, Lund.

Koch, R. 1967, *Grâce et liberté: Réflexion théologique sur Genèse I-XI*, Desclée, Paris.

Lacroix, X. 1992, *Le corps de chair: Les dimensions éthique, esthétique et spirituelle de l'amour*, Cerf, Paris.

Lega, C. 1991, *Manuale di Bioetica e Deontologia Medica*, Vita e Pensiero, Milan.

Leon-Dufour, X. 1981, *Dictionnaire de Théologie Biblique*, Cerf, Paris.

Lys, D. 1967, *La Chair dans l'Ancien Testament*, éd. Universiatires, Paris.

Macdonald, M. Y. 1991, 'Women in Body and Spirit: The Social Setting of 1 Corinthians 7', in *New Testament Studies*, vol. 36, pp. 161-181.

Mahmoud, M. 1977, *Du doute à la foi*, al-Shorouk, Beirut.

Mahmūd, M. 1989, *Al-Islām mā Huwa? (Qu'est que l'Islam)*, Dar al-Ma'ārif, Beirut.

Marcel, G. 1951, *Being and Having*, translated By K. Farrer, Beacon Press, Boston.

Masson, D. 1976, *Monothéisme Biblique et Monothéisme Coranique: Doctrines Comparées*, Desclée, Paris.

Mercatali, A. 1985, 'Antropologica filosofica', in *Antonianum*, vol. 68, 3rd ed., pp. 183-193.

Nachabeh, H. 1996, 'Transplantation des organs. La position de l'Islam', *Symposium de bioéthique*, Université Saint-Esprit Kaslik, Lebanon.

Penna, R. 1984, 'Annotazioni su amore e sessualità dall'Antico as Nuovo Testamento', in *Seminarium*, vol. 24, pp. 40-51.

Piana, G. 1990, 'Orientamenti di etica sessuale', in T. Goffi and G. Piana (eds), *Corso di morale: Ettica della personna* (2nd ed.), Queriniana, Brescia.

Piana, G. 1994, 'Sessualità', in L. Salvino and P. Salvatore (eds), *Dizionario di bioetica*, Edizioni Dehoniane Bologna-Instituto Siciliano di Bioetica, Bologna.

Pontifical Council for the Family 1996, *The Truth And Meaning Of Human Sexuality: Guidelines for Education within the Family*, Holy See, Rome.

Pontifical Council for Health Pastoral Care 1995, *Charter for Health Care Workers*, Holy See, Rome.

Reich, W.T. (ed.) 1978, *Encyclopaedia of Bioethics*, vol. 1, Simon and Schuster, New York.

Ratzinger, J. 1977, *Le Dieu de Jésus-Christ: Méditations sur Dieu-Trinité*, Fayard, Paris.

Robinson, J. A. T. 1962, *Le corps: Etude sur la théologie de Saint Paul*, Chalet, Paris.

Rocchetta, C. 1993, *Per una Teologia della corporeità*, Camilliane, Torino.

Rossi, G. 1992, 'Sessualità, matrimonio e famiglia', in L. Lorenzetti (ed.), *Trattato di etica teologica: Etica della personna* (2nd ed.), Edizioni Dehoniane Bologna, Bologna.

Sacred Congregation for Catholic Education 1984, *Educational Guidance In Human Love: Outlines for Sex Education*, Holy See, Rome.

Sacred Congregation for the Doctrine of Faith 1975, *Persona Humana: Declaration on Certain Questions Concerning Sexual Ethics*, Holy See, Rome.

Schweizer, E. 1965, 'Saarx, sarkikos, sarkinos', in G. Kittel (ed.), *Grande Lessico del Nuovo Testamento*, Paideia, Brescia, pp. 1268-1398.

Serour, G. I. 1996, 'Islam and the Four Principles', in G. Raanan (ed.), *Principles of Health Care Ethics*, John Wiley and Sons, New York.

Second Vatican Council 1965, *Gaudium et Spes (Pastoral Constitution On The Church In The Modern World)*, Holy See, Rome.

Seyyed, H. N. 1976, *Islamic Science: An Illustrated Study*, World of Islam Festival Publishing Company Ltd, England.

Sgreccia, E. 1994, *Manuale di Bioetica: Fondamenti ed etica biomedical. Vol. 1*, Vita e Pensiero, Milan.

Simonetti, N. 1994, 'Deontologia Medica,' in L. Salvino and P. Salvatore (eds), *Dizionario di bio*etica, Edizioni Dehoniane Bologna-Instituto Siciliano di Bioetica, Bologna.

Sioutti, J. E. 1994, *La medicine du prophète*, Dar al-Bouraq, Beirut.

Spinsanti, S. 1990, 'Salute, malattia, morte', in *Nuovo Dizionario di Teologia Morale*, Paoline, Milan.

Synode Diocésain de Suisse Romande 1975, 'Décisions sur mariage et famille', in *Documentation Catholique*, vol. 1671.

Talbi, M. and Bucaille, M. 1989, *Reflexions sue le Coran*, Seghers, Paris.

Théo Nouvelle Encyclopédie Catholique 1989, Droguet-Ardant, Fayard.

Thevenot, X. 1975, *Repères éthiques pour un monde nouveau*, Salvator, Mulhouse-France.

Tomiche, N. 1971, 'Femme', in *Encyclopédie de l'Islam*, vol. 2, pp. 452-457.

UNESCO 1981, *Universal Islamic Declaration of Human Rights*, 19 September 1981, Paris, http://www.alhewar.com/ISLAMDECL.html

Vidal, M. 1996, *Manuale di etica teologica: Morale dell'amore e della sessualita* (Part 2. 2nd ed.), Cittadella Editrice, Assisi.

Yaljin, M. 1973, *Al-Ittigāh al-ahlāqī fil-islām: Dirāsa mūqārana (L'Orientation morale dans l'Islam: Étude comparée)*, Al-Khangī, Egypt.

Yasin, M. N. 1996, *Abhāt fiqhīya fi qadāyā tubbīya mu'āsira (Recherche legislative dans des questions médicales contemporaines)*, Dar al-Nafa'is, Jordan.

About the Author

His Excellency Bishop Antoine-Charbel Tarabay, Bishop of the Maronite Eparchy of Australia is a monk and priest in the Lebanese Maronite Order, a religious order of the Maronite Catholic Church.

Born and raised in Tannourine, situated in the mountains of North Lebanon, Bishop Tarabay's lifelong vocation was perhaps inevitable having been raised to be both pious and thirsty for knowledge. Bishop Tarabay's birthland has been enriched by the heritage of the Maronite Catholic faith, which instilled a personal dedication that led him to make commit to his vocation in 1993 when he was ordained a priest in the Lebanese Maronite Order.

After completing his undergraduate studies in 1993, majoring in Theology at the University of the Holy Spirit in Kaslik, Lebanon, Bishop Tarabay moved to Italy to complete two Masters Degrees where he graduated with Honours [Moral Theology (1996) and Bioethics (1998)]. He also completed a Diploma in Human Rights Studies (1999) at the Institute of Human Rights in the Catholic University of Lyon, France, before returning to Rome to finish his Doctorate. In 1999, Bishop Tarabay was awarded a Doctorate of Moral Theology (Bioethics), from Academia Alfonsiana – Lateran University, after completing his thesis, *Bioéthique Catholique et Bioéthique Musulmane: étude d'éthique comparée en vue d'une bioéthique interreligieuse* ("Catholic and Islamic Bioethics: A Study in Comparative Ethics Envisaging an Inter-Religious Bioethics").

Bishop Tarabay's passion for education has seen him work at all levels, from primary to tertiary. His career in education started in 1999 as a Lecturer in Business Ethics and Bioethics at Holy Spirit University in Lebanon and as a Lecturer in Moral Theology at the Antonine University in Lebanon. In 2002, he was appointed Principal of St Charbel's Primary and Secondary College in Sydney, before returning to Lebanon in 2005 as the Director of Student Affairs at the University of the Holy Spirit. During his second post at that university, Bishop Tarabay also lectured in Bioethics.

In 2007, Bishop Tarabay returned to St Charbel's in Sydney, as the Rector. This post incorporated the role of Father Superior of St Charbel's Parish, College and Monastery. He has been an advocate of excellence in educational delivery and resources.

Bishop Tarabay's work was recognised by the Premier of New South Wales for his community service, receiving the Community Service Award (2004) and a Certificate of Commendation (2005).

A respected academic, Bishop Tarabay's first publication, *God, Nature and Person: Thoughts on the Foundations of Bioethics in Christianity and Islam*, will be the first volume of three.

Glossary

Anthropology – the study of humans, their origins, physical characteristics, institutions, religious beliefs, social relationships, and so on.

Basar – the human person in the corporeal state. The term is mentioned more than 270 times in the Old Testament. In the first instance, when referring to the human person, *basar* means *flesh*, namely the totality of the body. But more precisely, *basar* refers to the integrlity of the human being. It also indicates the material substance that forms the body, that is, the male body was formed from the silt of the earth, while the female was formed from the male body .

Bible – the Christian Sacred Scriptures, divided into two parts: the *Old Testament* and the *New Testament*. For Christians, the combination of the two Testaments comprises the "theological perspective" of the Bible,which is a; a deposit of revelation. The Bible was written by writers inspired by the Holy Spirit, to communicate and record the word of God. The Bible is both a sacred and human text , making it relevant to literature as well as to theology. In this study, we employ the 1990 edition of the New Jerusalem Bible .

Bioethics – that part of moral philosophy which determines whether it is licit or not to intervene in the life of man, particularly when related to the practice and development of medical and biological sciences.

Catechism of the Catholic Church – a summary of the Catholic doctrine of faith and morals. It is designed for use in catechesis, that is, education in the faith. Generally speaking, it imparts Catholic doctrine in an organic and systematic way, with a view to initiating the hearers into the fullness of Christian life.

Christology – theological interpretation of the person and work of Jesus Christ.

Corporeality – bodily or material nature or substance; physical existence.

Deontology – studies the difficulties of reconciling medical practice and social rules. It explores and identifies the rights and duties of the medical practitioner. It also studies the doctor's authority and its exercise according to the needs, requirements and expectations of individuals and the community, for the best interest and the greater good of the human being.

Epistemological – the branch of philosophy that studies the nature of knowledge, its presuppositions and foundations, and its extent and validity.

Fiqh – Islamic academics or the *Fuqaha'* Scholars, have created the *Fiqh* manuals using a method of deduction and interpretation. The *Fiqh* is the Islamic judicial system that covers the norms that govern the relationships between individuals and their relationship with God. The *fatwa-s* issued by religious groups are subsequently added to the *Fiqh* manuals. The *fatwa-s* are circulated by radio, television and newspaper media, and are responses to answers raised by the general public or state authorities, and clarify conduct and practices as appropriate for the Islamic religion. *Fatwa-s* are more often than not, widely published and broadcast.

Hadith – the words, the acts, the explicit and implicit endorsements are attributed to Muhammad, and as recorded in the texts of the *Hadith*.

Ishsha – the identity of woman as formed concurrently with the identity of man, *ish*.

Koran – this document is the primary source of faith and ethics for all Muslims. It is the revelation passed on by Allah to Muhammad from the year 610 until his death in 632. It is believed that Allah Himself, not Muhammad, is the author of Koran. The current text of the Koran was written some 15 to 20 years after Muhammad's death, and consists of 114 *suras* or chapters in no chronological order. The *suras* are organised in a descending order according to their length, resulting in a sudden switch from one topic to the next. Each section of the Koran is said to have been revealed in response to certain situations, or to answer questions that were asked of Muhammad. This is said to be the case for the *asbab al-nazul* revelation, which helps to explain Koranic text but is not necessarily included in the Koran. For the purposes of this study, the English translation of the Koran by Mohammed Marmaduke Pickthall (1930) is used.

Leb / Lebab – Hebrew for the "heart". These terms are mentioned over 860 times in the Old Testament, and refer to the centre of activity of 'man,' his faculties of intelligence, and thus indicate the totality of the human person capable of thinking and choosing freely. The heart of 'man' is not merely a bodily organ; it qualifies 'man' himself. It characterises the human person in both his emotive and physical realities. The heart is also considered to be the origin of evil, for sin against the divine will of God is not attributed not to the body but to the heart.

Lordship – stewardship, especially in the sense of a function which combines both authority over and responsibility towards a charge.

Magisterium – the written teachings and attitude of the Catholic Church, as they relate to the theology and the everyday practices of all Christians. Etymologically, the Magisterium refers to the teachings of an expert. More specifically, it refers to the teachings of an authority. As such, the term "Magisterium" has been applied by the Catholic tradition to the teachings of God, Christ, the Apostles and the teaching authorities of the Church. The term was first applied in 1837 by Gregory XVI, delegating those within the Church with the authority to teach. Magisterium in the Catholic Church is therefore, an authority , and is based on processes that have gradually developed throughout history. It has become the criterion of the revealed truth entrusted to the Church, not only to itself as an authority, but also for its connection to the *'sensus fidei'* (sense of faith) of God's people. In the customary sense, the Magisterium does not designate a doctoral authority but rather refers to those who are its subjects or authors, that is, the Pope and the Episcopal body.

'Man'/Woman – a divine creation in Catholicism and Islam. 'Man' in the theological tradition of the monotheistic religions, is *the masterpiece of the creation*. Biblical theology regards 'man' as being exclusively created in the image of God, as man and woman who are equal in dignity. Man in Islam, is a privileged being that was made by the hands of the Creator, as Viceroy of the universe. In Islam, woman is not equal to man, given her dependence on him. The Catholic position is one of equal value and dignity, and co- dependence.

Mediate Animation – the view that the soul enters the new human person immediately at the moment of conception is known as "immediate animation". That it enters at some point after conception (without necessarily defining when) is known as "mediate animation"

Minimalism – a simple religious framework based on the principle that the more complex the set of beliefs, the more likely it is to reflect wrong assumptions from the various and often unknown people who have contributed to it. This does not mean that another religion is necessarily wrong. It is a framework rather than a religion because it sees religion as being about the personal relationship with the Divine, so the minimalist framework aims to provide some uncluttered space for that personal relationship to develop.

Monotheistic Religions – the belief in a single God, as opposed to polytheism (the belief in multiple gods). Monotheism is chiefly represented in our culture by three religions – Judaism, Christianity and Islam. These religions preach the existence of a sole Supreme Being who is absolute, infinite, spiritual and personal, Creator of the world and 'man' whilst being separate from them. Their faith is based on the revelation of God through His own word. For Jews, the word of God is conveyed in the Torah; for Christians, aside from the Bible, the word of God is personified in Jesus Christ . For followers of Islam, the Koran is the transcript of the word of Allah received by Mohammed.

Neotestamentary – relating to the New Testament .

Nihilism – the belief that all values are baseless, and often that no absolute truth can be known or communicated. It is often associated with extreme pessimism and a radical skepticism that condemns existence as meaningless. A true nihilist would believe in nothing, have no loyalties, and no purpose other than, perhaps, an impulse to destroy the meaningless. Its corrosive effects would eventually destroy all moral, religious, and metaphysical convictions and precipitate the greatest crisis in human history.

Parousia – the second coming of Jesus Christ.

Personalist Bioethics – in Catholicism is based on the premise that the human being is perceived as an end, not a means. The dignity, value and autonomy of every person – man and woman – represent a characteristic element of Catholic anthropology, and, thus considered, is the main reason for the conception of a personalist approach to bioethics. With that in mind, equality between man and woman in Islam is inconceivable and even impossible. Indeed, a personalist bioethical approach is particularly impossible in the Islamic world.

Pneuma – the spirit of 'man,' as opposed to his flesh *(sarx)*, in which 'man' in his totality is left to make choices according to either his *pneuma* or *sarx*.

Sarx – refers to the flesh associated with the creation. The *sarx* is characterised by existence as a perishable, weak and mortal being that is distanced from God, and has sinned in Adam and Eve. According to St Paul, *sarx* does not indicate a part of the human person, but rather nominates the person as a whole in his visible reality or, more frequently, in his fragility and morality.

Seigniory – see "Lordship" above.

Shari'a – collection of Islamic teachings, that are not attributed to a single authority or entity, and have not been declared as official doctrine. The *Shari'a* is comprised of two components: the *Sunna* or the tradition of Muhammad, and the *Fiqh* jurisprudence manuals. In the context of this study, the term *Shari'a* refers to any of the Isalmic schools of thought composing the *Shari'a*. It will not allow the discussion to focus on specific themes or topics that are not necessarily covered by either of the components in the *Shari'a*. As such, any theme or topic in either of the sources of the *Shari'a* will be regarded as an authoritative the Islamic teaching. Overall, the *Shari'a* is a compilation of the instructions that regulate daily life, to which every good Muslim must adhere. Except in the areas of worship, religious rites and moral codes, the *Shari'a* is not a rigid or set text.

Soma – the Greek word for "body", used to refer to 'man' as part of the creation, and the sinful human condition, while still acknowledging the value of his being, because he was created by God and owes his existence to Him. In general, *soma* implies a positive concept of the body. It is no longer the flesh (*sarx*) of passion, sin and death, but the baptised body to be offered to God. *Soma* then, is not equivalent to *sarx*, but to *basar*, thus to 'man' in his entirety, whether in his internal structure or visible form.

Subsidiarity – the teaching of the Church, found especially in its social doctrine, that so far as it is both possible and appropriate, decisions should be made by the person or entity who must implement that decision. It is opposed to central planning, which too often removes from subordinates (hence the name of the principle) the right to make decisions which affect them directly. It is not that no central planning should ever be undertaken, but that where possible, the relevant 'subordinate" should be left freedom of action and choice.

Veterotestamentary – relating to the writings of the Old Testament.

www.ingramcontent.com/pod-product-compliance
Ingram Content Group UK Ltd.
Pitfield, Milton Keynes, MK11 3LW, UK
UKHW041414180426
11947UKWH00007B/136